CERVICAL SMEAR TEST

What every woman should know

Albert Singer, FRCOG
and
Dr Anne Szarewski

Recommended by the Family Planning Association

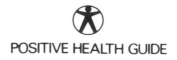

POSITIVE HEALTH GUIDE

©Albert Singer and Anne Marie Szarewski 1988

First published in 1988 by
Macdonald Optima, a division of
Macdonald & Co. (Publishers) Ltd
Reprinted 1989

A member of Maxwell Pergamon Publishing Corporation plc

British Library Cataloguing in Publication Data
Singer, Albert
    Cervical smear test
    1. Women. Uterus. Cervix. Lesions –
    Illustrations – For colposcopy
    I. Title   II. Szarewski, Anne III. Series
    618.1'4
    ISBN 0-356-15065-8

Macdonald & Co. (Publishers) Ltd
66–73 Shoe Lane
London EC4P 4AB

Photoset in 11pt Times by ᴦᴀTek Art Limited, Croydon, Surrey

Printed and bound in Great Britain at the University Press, Cambridge

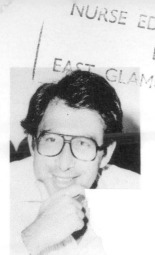

Albert Singer FRCOG, has been Consultant Obstetrician and Gynaecologist at the Whittington and Royal Northern Hospitals since 1980. He heads one of the largest colposcopy and oncology clinics in Europe, and an active research team which has a particular interest in using lasers in the treatment of precancers.

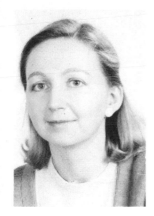

Anne Szarewski DRCOG, trained initially at the Middlesex Hospital Medical School, London and then in Obstetrics and Gynaecology at the Royal Northern and Whittington Hospitals. She currently works as a Family Planning Doctor at a Well Woman clinic, as a clinical assistant in genito-urinary medicine at St Thomas's Hospital, London and as a clinical assistant in colposcopy at the Royal Northern.

CONTENTS

ACKNOWLEDGMENTS

Thanks are due to the following for their help: Maggie Raynor for the line illustrations; National Testing Laboratories Processing (UK) for the cervicography photographs; Sharplan Lasers (Europe) Ltd; Middlesex Hospital Photographic Department; Hugh Oliff; Medscand (Sweden) and D. H. Colgate Medical Ltd. (Windsor, Berks), manufacturers of the Cytobrush; Steriseal Ltd, manufacturers of the Cervex; Zefa picture library for the cover photograph.

PREFACE

It is still a sad fact that the majority of women who develop cervical cancer have never had a smear. We believe that at least part of the reason for this is a combination of ignorance – of their need to be tested – and fear of both the test itself and of what might follow.

There is also a sizeable and growing number of women who find they have an abnormal smear, and are unsure of what that means, how they got it and what will happen to them.

Women often feel that doctors are too busy to answer their questions, so they do not ask. Our aim, in writing this book, is to provide answers to those questions. In this way, we hope to dispel at least some of these fears and uncertainties. There are questions to which there are no easy answers at present; however, we hope we can give an insight into the reasoning behind what sometimes appear to be conflicting and contradictory medical opinions.

Although the book is primarily aimed at women, we hope that men will also find it useful. Cervical cancer is a sexually transmitted disease, and should therefore be a matter of concern for both partners.

We would like to thank Dr Gary Patou for his expert advice and help in the preparation of Chapters 7 and 8. We would also like to thank our editor, Harriet Griffey, for her encouragement and support throughout the writing of this book.

1
—

THE CERVIX AND THE SMEAR TEST

WHAT IS THE CERVIX?

The cervix is just a name given to the lower part of the uterus (womb). As you can see from the diagrams on pages 2 and 3, the womb is shaped rather like an upside-down pear; the wide part is called the body and the narrow part is the cervix. Another way of describing it would be as a head and neck; obviously, the wide part is the 'head', while the cervix corresponds with the 'neck'. So, if you hear anyone talking about the 'neck of the womb', they mean the cervix.

Seen face on, the cervix looks round, with a hole in the middle. In a woman who has not had children, or who has had them by Caesarean section, the hole, or external os as it is called, is perfectly round. During childbirth the hole is stretched a great deal, to allow the baby to come through. Afterwards it does not go back to its original shape and size; it tends to be more slit-shaped, and wider than before.

The cervix also has an internal os, which is a tight band of muscle just behind the external os. This muscle is very important in pregnancy as it prevents the growing baby from falling out of the womb, or miscarrying. The internal os stays tightly shut until a woman actually begins labour, when it very gradually stretches open. It is the 'body' of the uterus which enlarges during the nine months of pregnancy, and which contains and nourishes the baby.

The hole in the cervix has another function – letting substances pass in and out of the womb. For example, when

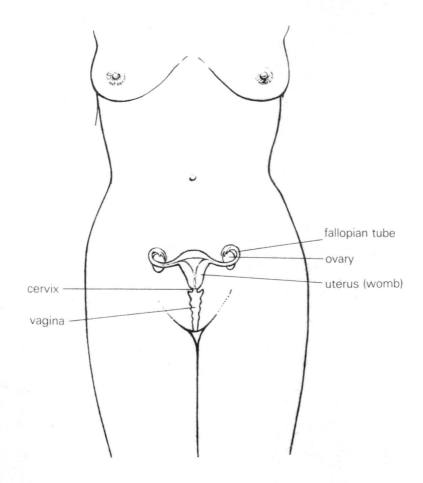

Female reproductive organs.

you have a period the blood comes out through the cervix. When you have sex, sperm reach the ovary via the hole in the cervix. Of course, nasty things such as infections can also get in through this hole.

THE CERVIX UNDER THE MICROSCOPE

Since the two parts of the uterus have different functions, it is not surprising that they are made up of different types of cells.

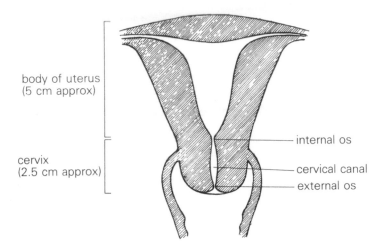

body of uterus
(5 cm approx)

cervix
(2.5 cm approx)

internal os

cervical canal

external os

Uterus and cervix.

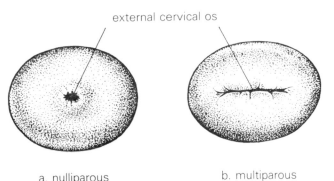

external cervical os

a. nulliparous
(i.e. a woman who has
not had children)

b. multiparous
(i.e. a woman who
has had children)

View of the cervix, face on.

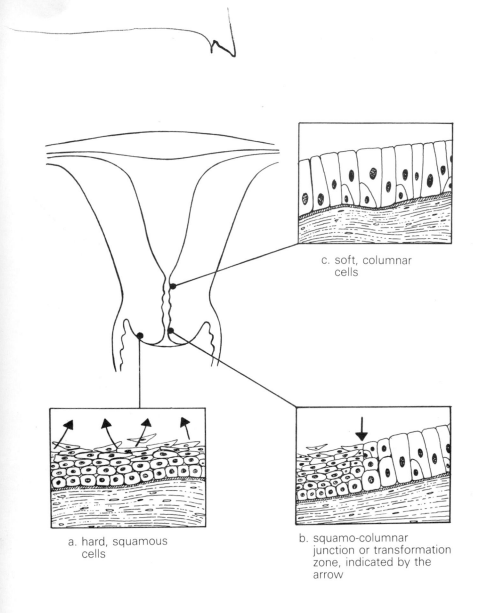

c. soft, columnar
cells

a. hard, squamous
cells

b. squamo-columnar
junction or transformation
zone, indicated by the
arrow

Cells of the cervix and uterus.

Cells are the building blocks from which all living things are made, and have a variety of shapes, sizes and functions. Inside the body of the uterus there are soft columnar (meaning tall and narrow) cells. They have a good blood supply – this is why, when part of the lining comes away every month, you bleed, i.e. have a period.

The cervix is exposed to the outside world via the vagina (front passage). Because they can expect some rough treatment, the cells on the outside surfaces of the vagina and cervix are hard squamous (flat) cells, which don't have such a good blood supply (otherwise every time you make love you would bleed). These tough squamous cells are separated from the deeper, connective tissues, containing blood vessels and glands, by a continuous layer of cells called the basement membrane. This is a physical barrier between the outer and inner layers of cells, and becomes very important when we look at the development and treatment of cervical cancer in Chapter 6.

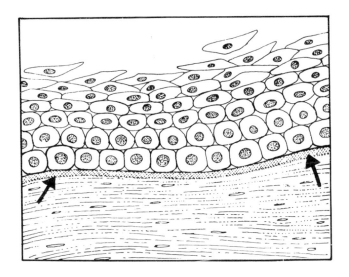

Squamous layer of cells separated from the connective tissue by the basement membrane (indicated by arrows).

Under a microscope, the surface of the cervix is not a smooth line but, rather like the coastline on a map, is irregular, with many folds. Sometimes these crypts, as they are called, get blocked off, rather like a lagoon which becomes a lake. When this happens, they look like little cysts on the surface of the cervix, and are called Nabothian follicles, after the doctor who first noticed them.

Since the body of the uterus and the cervix are not separated by a physical space (there is no gap between them in the uterus), there has to be an area where the two types of cells (i.e. squamous and columnar) are next to and, to some extent, mixed in with one another. This is called the squamo-columnar junction – see figure on page 4. You will hear much more about this important area in Chapter 3, because this is where abnormal cells first appear. However, before we get too involved in difficult biology, let's look at the cervical smear and why it is so important.

WHAT IS A CERVICAL SMEAR?

Cervical cancer is a totally preventable disease. Despite this fact, over 2,000 women in England and Wales alone die of it every year. The majority of them die because they have never had a cervical smear – a fact which is particularly tragic when you think how simple and quick the test is.

A cervical smear (also called a Pap test or Papanicolaou smear) is a screening test for cervical cancer and for the early cell changes which may eventually lead to cervical cancer. It is important to stress here that the whole point of a screening test is to pick up early changes *before* you have any symptoms. The fact that you feel quite well and have not noticed anything unusual makes no difference; you should still have a smear.

Any woman who has *ever* had sex should have regular smears. In Chapters 7 and 8 we will be looking in detail at the possible causes of cervical cancer, but the one thing which stands out is that they are all related in some way to sex.

Taking a smear involves nothing more than having a full vaginal examination. You are asked to lie on a couch and an instrument called a speculum is gently inserted into the vagina (front passage). This should not be painful, though if you are very tense it can be uncomfortable. If you know you are likely

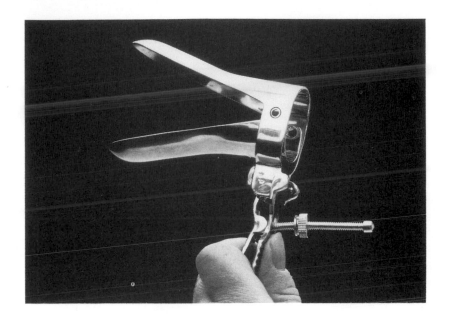

An open speculum.

to be tense and anxious, try and prepare yourself beforehand; obviously, don't plan to have your smear on a day when you have other stressful things to cope with. Some women find it helpful to have a friend with them, at least in the waiting room.

The speculum is necessary because the doctor or nurse has to be able to see your cervix in order to take the smear accurately. A sample taken from the wrong place is useless, and only results in a repeat performance. When the speculum is opened, it pushes apart the walls of the vagina, allowing the cervix to be seen.

A spatula is then gently wiped across the cervix in order to collect some of the loose cells. There are many different types of spatula available nowadays; some are made of wood, some of plastic, and they can also vary in shape. It is important the smear samples come from the right areas (see Chapter 2). Unfortunately, the most important area is often hidden deep in the cervical canal, which is why the newer spatulas have a more pointed end, and also why the cytobrush was developed. The cytobrush fits snugly into the cervical canal and has

7

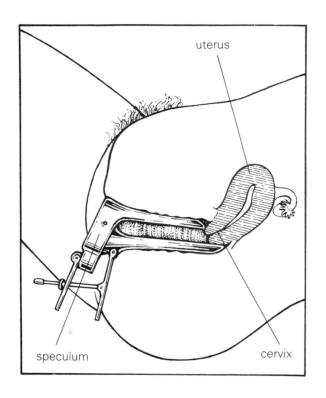

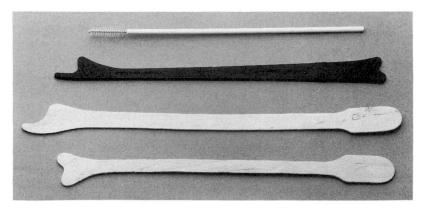

Speculum in place during a vaginal examination.

From top to bottom:
Cytobrush   Aylesbury spatula
Lerners spatula   Ayres' spatula

8

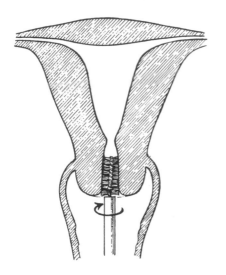

a. Cytobrush

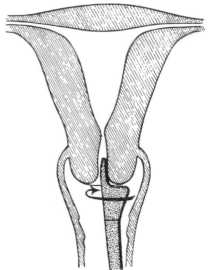

b. Lerners spatula

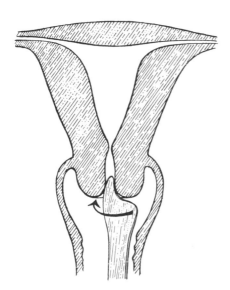

c. Aylesbury spatula

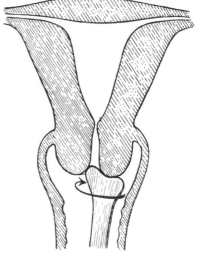

d. Ayres' spatula

Using the spatula or cytobrush.

proved the most efficient method to date. It does tend to cause a little bleeding, so don't panic if you find you are spotting a little after having a smear.

After the smear has been taken the speculum is removed and, as far as you are concerned, the whole thing is over. From beginning to end it takes less than five minutes.

WHAT HAPPENS TO THE SMEAR?

Once it has been removed, the spatula or brush is wiped on a microscope slide, transferring the cells onto the slide, and the cells are preserved by pouring on an alcohol solution. Once this has been done, the smear will keep for years. The slide is then sent to a special laboratory where the cells are examined very carefully under a microscope by trained technicians and doctors called cytologists. (Cytology just means the study of cells; 'cyto' means 'cell' in Greek, and anything 'ology' means 'the study of'. Since Greek is very rarely taught in schools nowadays, doctors have just as much trouble with all this as you do!) Each slide has to be looked at in turn and any slide which shows an abnormality under the microscope is double checked, so the process is quite time consuming.

Finally, a report is sent back to the clinic. The report is usually written on the original smear form, and is partly standardised. One of the purposes of this book is to help you to understand the way in which a smear result is reported – not least because so much anxiety is caused by women reading smear reports which are, in fact, quite normal!

EXPLAINING THE CERVICAL SMEAR FORM

The illustration shows the most commonly used smear form. As you can see, the left-hand side gives your personal details, such as name, address, date of birth, as well as your clinic number, the doctor and clinic where it was taken, and the name and address of your GP. Those of you wondering about section 07 may be interested to know that married women are still classed under their husbands' occupation for statistical purposes. Social-class statistics are based on occupation,

| OR CLINIC CASE REFERENCE NO | 02 | 249810 | | ADDRESS (TOWN) OF LABORATORY | | | | |

			SERIAL NO.			

		DATE OF	DAY	MTH	YR
SURNAME	CLARKE	MAIDEN NAME	15 THIS TEST	15	11	87
FIRST NAMES	ANNE		16 LMP (1st day)	26	10	87
FULL POSTAL ADDRESS			17 LAST TEST			84
			18 NO PREVIOUS TEST (put x)			

12 MARITAL STATE
Single ①
Married 2
Widowed/ 2
Divorced 3

13 PREGNANCIES
Total births ⊘ (live and still)
Total of ⊘ abortions and miscarriages

14 CONDITION
Pregnant 1
Post-natal 2 (under 12 weeks)
IUCD fitted 16
On oral ④ contraceptive
On other 8 hormone (specify in Box 21)

20 APPEARANCE OF CERVIX
Normal ①
Eroded 2
Cervicitis 4
Polyp 8
Malignant 16

03

A	JONES	IF HOSPITAL STATE:-
NAME AND ADDRESS OF SENDER IF NOT GP		CONSULTANT
		WARD
		HOSPITAL

Fold for B

19 SYMPTOMS
Discharge 1   Post-menopausal 8 bleeding
Post-coital bleeding 2   Other symptoms 16 (Specify in Box 21)
Inter-menstrual bleeding 4

21 CLINICAL DATA (PREVIOUS TREATMENT INCLUDING RADIO THERAPY/CHEMOTHERAPY)

Fold

04 DATE OF BIRTH	DAY 1	MONTH 2	YEAR
Fold for A		04	57

06	GP 1	HOSPITAL 4	06 NHS NO
SOURCE OF SMEAR	AHA 2 Other 5	FP CLINIC ③	

07 HUSBAND'S OCCUPATION (patient's if unmarried) also state if Manager, Foreman or other
Production Assr.

22 CYTOLOGY REPORT

signature

08

B	
NAME AND ADDRESS OF GP	

23 EVIDENCE OF NEOPLASIA CYTOLOGICAL PATTERN SUGGESTS:
Inadequate specimen 1
Negative ②
Mild dysplasia 3
Severe dysplasia/ 4 carcinoma-in-situ
Carcinoma-in- 5 situ/? invasive
? Glandular neoplasia 6

24 INFLAMMATION
Severe 1 Inflammatory Change
Trichomonas 2
Candida 4
Viral 8

26 FURTHER INVESTIGATION SUGGESTED
Repeat smear
in ____ months 1 or after treatment
Colposcopy 16
Cervical biopsy 4
Uterine curettage 8

Signature ____ date

Fold

09 SPECIMEN TYPE	Cervical ①	Vaginal scrape 2	Cyto pipette 4	Other (specify) 8	LOCAL CODES	26	27	28	29	30

Request/Report/Recall Form for Cervical or Vaginal Cytology – SENDER's COPY

11

Completed smear form.

which is why this is included on the form (see Chapter 7 for more explanation).

The upper part of the right-hand section deals mainly with your medical history, e.g. number of pregnancies, type of contraception, date of your last period (LMP) and so on. These may be relevant for the cytologists as they may influence the appearance of the cells. Just as an example, cells look quite different at different times of the menstrual cycle, so the date of the last period is therefore important. There is a section (21) for your doctor/nurse to fill in if there are any other important details; for example, if you have had an abnormal smear before.

23 EVIDENCE OF NEOPLASIA CYTOLOGICAL PATTERN SUGGESTS		24 INFLAMMATION		25 FURTHER INVESTIGATION SUGGESTED	
Inadequate specimen	1	Severe Inflammatory Change	1	Repeat smear	
Negative	2	Trichomonas	2	in months	1
Mild dysplasia	3			or after treatment	2
Severe dysplasia/ carcinoma-in-situ	4	Candida	4	Colposcopy 16	
Carcinoma-in-situ/? invasive	5	Viral	8	Cervical biopsy	4
? Glandular neoplasia	6	Signature		Uterine curettage 8	
				date	

Smear form result showing inadequate specimen.

The bottom right-hand section gives the smear report. As you can see, in sections 23, 24 and 25 there are numbers corresponding to the gradings. So, for example, if your smear is normal (negative) there will be a circle round number 2 in section 23. If the quality of the smear was not good enough, number 1 (inadequate specimen) in section 23 will be circled – this means the smear will have to be repeated. We will be discussing the rest of the classifications in section 23 in the next chapter.

Section 24 deals mainly with infections which can show up on a smear. For example, if candida (thrush, yeast infection) is seen on the slide, number 4 will be circled. This is discussed further in Chapter 3.

12

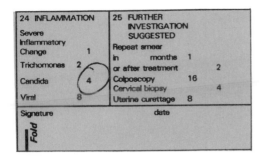

24 INFLAMMATION	25 FURTHER INVESTIGATION SUGGESTED	
Severe Inflammatory Change	Repeat smear	
1	in months 1	
Trichomonas 2	or after treatment	2
Candida 4	Colposcopy 16	
	Cervical biopsy	4
Viral 8	Uterine curettage 8	
Signature	date	

Smear form result showing candida.

Section 22 is a space in which the cytologists can write any extra comments about that particular smear, and it is these comments which usually cause the most anxiety and misunderstanding. By far the commonest are 'endocervical cells seen' or 'endocervical cells not seen'; these terms are explained in Chapter 3. Sometimes the remarks are so technical that even your doctor may find it difficult to understand them; however, by the time you have finished this book you will at least be able to make sense of the most common and most important ones.

In section 25 the cytologists suggest what should be done in the light of the smear result. For example, if the smear is normal they will write in when the next one should be taken; this will vary according to your geographical area, the current government guidelines, and the opinion of the cytologists (see Chapter 9). Your doctor, though, may have reason not to follow the recommendation; if you are confused, don't

24 INFLAMMATION	25 FURTHER INVESTIGATION SUGGESTED	
Severe Inflammatory Change	Repeat smear	
1	in 12 months 1	
Trichomonas 2	or after treatment	2
Candida 4	Colposcopy 16	
	Cervical biopsy	4
Viral 8	Uterine curettage 8	
Signature	date	

Smear form result recommending a repeat test in 12 months.

hesitate to ask what is happening, and why.

Probably the most important area of the form from your point of view is section 23, which tells you whether you have a negative or a positive smear. So what is a positive smear? The next chapter explains this.

2

THE POSITIVE SMEAR

WHAT IS A POSITIVE SMEAR?

A 'positive' smear is one which is not negative. That may sound like an insult to your intelligence, but what we are trying to stress here is that this term is used to describe several different types and stages of abnormality. A positive smear can therefore can mean anything, from something serious to the very mildest abnormality. It is thus an alarming and not very useful phrase.

ABNORMAL CHANGES

To understand the different types of abnormality that show up on smears, we must go back to our discussion of columnar and squamous cells (see Chapter 1). Around the cervical canal there is a junction point, where the soft columnar cells stop and the hard squamous cells begin. This is called the squamo-columnar junction. In this area, the soft columnar cells gradually adapt and change into squamous cells. This is a normal process and is called squamous metaplasia (metaplasia just means a change, or transformation). The actual area in which this change, or transformation, is taking place is called the transformation *zone*. (You can tell this is a relatively recent concept; it wasn't named in Greek.) Thus, the cells on a normal cervix are distributed as shown in the illustration over the page. The most important cells are the ones which are in the process of change; these are the ones which can potentially change into the wrong kind of cells and become cancer cells.

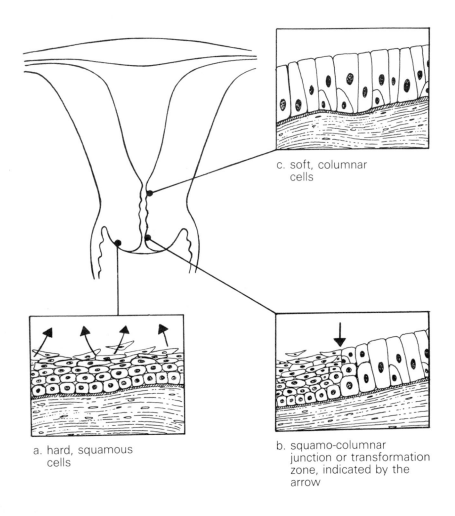

c. soft, columnar
cells

a. hard, squamous
cells

b. squamo-columnar
junction or transformation
zone, indicated by the
arrow

Cells of the cervix and uterus.

23 EVIDENCE OF NEOPLASIA CYTOLOGICAL PATTERN SUGGESTS:		24 INFLAMMATION		25 FURTHER INVESTIGATION SUGGESTED	
Inadequate specimen	1	Severe Inflammatory Change	1	Repeat smear in months	1
Negative	2	Trichomonas	2	or after treatment	2
Mild dysplasia	(3)	Candida	4	Colposcopy	16
Severe dysplasia/ carcinoma-in-situ	4			Cervical biopsy	4
Carcinoma-in-situ/? invasive	5	Viral	8	Uterine curettage	8
? Glandular neoplasia	6	Signature		date	

Smear form result showing mild dysplasia.

The first thing to say is that this change is a very slow process. However, very early changes in the cells can be seen under a microscope. Cells undergoing abnormal changes are called dysplastic cells ('dys' in Greek means 'bad' or 'abnormal', and 'plasia' means 'change'). At first the changes are slight and this is called 'mild dysplasia', i.e. mild abnormal change. If this happens to you, section 23 of your smear form will be marked as in the illustration above. If the cells carry on changing abnormally then, with time, they show more marked changes under the microscope; this is called moderate dysplasia. There is no category in which to fit this on the smear form,

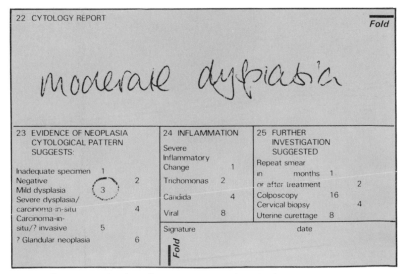

22 CYTOLOGY REPORT					*Fold*

moderate dysplasia (handwritten)

23 EVIDENCE OF NEOPLASIA CYTOLOGICAL PATTERN SUGGESTS:		24 INFLAMMATION		25 FURTHER INVESTIGATION SUGGESTED	
Inadequate specimen	1	Severe Inflammatory Change	1	Repeat smear in months	1
Negative	2	Trichomonas	2	or after treatment	2
Mild dysplasia	(3)	Candida	4	Colposcopy	16
Severe dysplasia/ carcinoma-in-situ	4			Cervical biopsy	4
Carcinoma-in-situ/? invasive	5	Viral	8	Uterine curettage	8
? Glandular neoplasia	6	Signature		date	

Smear form result showing moderate dysplasia.

23 EVIDENCE OF NEOPLASIA CYTOLOGICAL PATTERN SUGGESTS		24 INFLAMMATION		25 FURTHER INVESTIGATION SUGGESTED	
Inadequate specimen	1	Severe Inflammatory Change	1	Repeat smear in months	1
Negative	2	Trichomonas	2	or after treatment	2
Mild dysplasia	3	Candida	4	Colposcopy	16
Severe dysplasia/ carcinoma-in-situ	4	Viral	8	Cervical biopsy	4
Carcinoma-in-situ/? invasive	5			Uterine curettage	8
? Glandular neoplasia	6	Signature date			

Smear form result showing severe dysplasia.

so the cytologists usually cross out 'mild' and replace it with 'moderate', as in the illustration at the bottom of page 17. If the change becomes greater still it is called severe dysplasia (severe abnormal change).

A slightly newer classification refers to the changes in terms of dyskaryosis ('dys' means 'bad' or 'abnormal' as before, and 'karyon' means 'nucleus'). This is because the most important changes actually relate mainly to the nucleus of the cell. Thus, mild dysplasia becomes mild dyskaryosis, moderate dysplasia becomes moderate dyskaryosis, and severe dysplasia becomes severe dyskaryosis. The terms dysplasia and dyskaryosis are often used interchangeably.

You are bound to have noticed the nasty phrase 'carcinoma in situ' in the illustration. This is a very bad phrase, and doctors try not to use it any more. It means, literally, 'cancer which has not spread' ('in situ' is Latin for 'in the original place, or site'). This refers to the fact that in the smear in question, although there are many cells which show severe dysplasia, they have not penetrated the basement membrane (see Chapter 1) and therefore there is no sign of an actual invasive cancer. The reason that 'carcinoma in situ' is such a bad phrase is that it is so emotive, whereas in reality this abnormality is very simply and completely curable, just like the earlier forms of dysplasia.

Now it may have occurred to you that the examination of loose cells scraped off the cervix for a smear test will not tell the cytologist how they are related to the basement membrane. However, there is a subtle difference between the cells showing severe dysplasia and carcinoma in situ, which a cytologist can recognise.

At this point, it's important to stress and remember that *none* of the changes we have talked about so far are in fact cancer. They are merely abnormal cells which, given enough time (i.e. years), have the *potential* to become cancer. For this reason, you may see these cells being referred to as pre-cancer cells, meaning cells that appear before cancer. The whole point of the smear test is that cells can be identified while they are still in a pre-cancerous stage and then got rid of simply and easily, before they ever become dangerous.

THE CIN CLASSIFICATION

Just as you thought you were beginning to understand about dysplasia and cell changes, there is another system of classification to confuse you all over again! In fact it is a more logical system and not that difficult to follow.

CIN stands for cervical intra-epithelial neoplasia. 'Neoplasia' means 'new change' (neo = new, plasia = change), and 'intra-epithelial' means 'in the outer cell layer' ('intra' just means 'in' and 'epithelial' means 'that which covers the surface': they got so carried away with this that both Latin and Greek are thrown in). And 'cervical' simply means 'of the cervix'. So, in summary, CIN just means 'new changes in the outer cell layers of the cervix'.

Once you've grasped the initial concept, the rest is easy:
CIN grade 1 is the same as mild dysplasia or mild dyskaryosis.
CIN grade 2 is moderate dysplasia or moderate dyskaryosis.
And CIN grade 3 is severe dysplasia or severe dyskaryosis.

Remember that if your smear shows any of these grades of abnormality, you do *not* have cancer. However, because we know that these cells *can* progress to become cancer – despite the fact that this takes place very slowly – there is no point waiting for it to happen.

I HAVE A POSITIVE SMEAR. WHAT NEXT?

Firstly, DON'T PANIC! Remember, a positive smear could mean just the very first stage of abnormality (mild dysplasia). So, if you receive a letter saying your smear is abnormal, the first thing you need to do is find out exactly what it has shown. Make an appointment to see your doctor and discuss it with him or her. Don't be frightened to ask questions. There is no reason why you should not be shown your smear report form, so that you can see it with your own eyes. Women often feel something is being kept from them if they are not shown the report; in fact, very often, the doctor is simply worried that the technical terms will be frightening and incomprehensible. After reading this book, you should be in a good position to make sense of them.

Tens of thousands of women have a positive smear every year; you will not be alone. You almost certainly already know someone who has been through the experience; ask your friends. There are both good and bad sides to this. It may be reassuring to talk to a friend who has been through it all, who tells you it was not so dreadful, for whom everything turned out all right. Unfortunately, the people with the most to say are often the ones for whom everything went wrong; they may be in the minority, but their's are the stories that stick in the mind. As an analogy, remember that thousands of aeroplanes carry people safely to their destinations every day, but it is only when there is a disaster that you see reports in the newspapers. Listen, but try to keep an open mind.

So, the first thing to do is to establish what grade of abnormality your smear has shown. You may notice on your smear form that a course of action has been suggested in section 25. If your smear has shown any degree of dysplasia, colposcopy (number 16) will be recommended. Colposcopy is simply a way of looking more closely at the cervix ('colpos' means 'vagina' and 'oscopy' means 'to look at or through', i.e.

23 EVIDENCE OF NEOPLASIA CYTOLOGICAL PATTERN SUGGESTS:		24 INFLAMMATION		25 FURTHER INVESTIGATION SUGGESTED	
		Severe Inflammatory Change	1	Repeat smear in months	1
Inadequate specimen	1	Trichomonas	2	or after treatment	2
Negative	2			Colposcopy 16	
Mild dysplasia	3	Candida	4	Cervical biopsy	4
Severe dysplasia/ carcinoma-in-situ	4	Viral	8	Uterine curettage	8
Carcinoma-in-situ/? invasive	5	Signature		date	
? Glandular neoplasia	6	*Fold*			

Smear form result recommending colposcopy.

20

to look through the vagina at the cervix). It will be described in detail in Chapter 4.

Colposcopy is a relatively new technique and unfortunately there are, as yet, not enough doctors who know how to do it. As a service, it is also quite expensive to set up, mainly because the instruments are expensive. All this adds up to the inevitable long waiting lists. In some parts of Britain, women are having to wait several months for their appointment. Obviously, this causes an enormous amount of anxiety. No amount of reassurance will stop a woman worrying while she is waiting to be seen. If your smear shows moderate or severe dysplasia, you will be high up on the waiting list and you should not wait more than a few weeks to be seen. Bear in mind that the cell changes take a very long time (usually years) so a few more weeks are unlikely to make any difference.

Things are more complicated if your smear report shows a less severe abnormality, for example 'mild dysplasia'. In the past, nothing was done about these, other than repeating the smear every six months and waiting for it either to improve on its own or get worse. However, there are a number of problems with this approach. Firstly, it has been shown that the majority don't improve, i.e. they won't go away if we ignore them. Secondly, the smear is only a marker of abnormality; it should not be considered to be 100 per cent accurate. So, while a certain number of abnormal smears turn out to be false alarms, a number of women will have abnormalities which are in fact more severe than their smears suggest. About a third of smears which show only mild dysplasia actually turn out to be moderate or severe dysplasia when the woman has a colposcopy. So, really, any degree of abnormality should be looked at more closely, with the colposcope.

There is a major problem with this approach, however. In the United Kingdom, at least, the resources simply aren't there. If every woman was referred for a colposcopy after one abnormal smear, the clinics would be flooded with referrals and the waiting lists would become endless. For this reason, there are many areas where the policy continues to be one of repeating the smears. A more reasonable compromise in these circumstances is to repeat the smear once: if it is still abnormal, the woman is then referred for colposcopy; if it is

21

normal, she has yearly smears thereafter.

Cervicography is another technique which may help considerably with these problems in the future. It is described in Chapter 11.

And what should you do if you find that you are not being offered a colposcopy, despite having had several abnormal smears? The simple answer is make an appointment to see your doctor and discuss the problem with him or her. It can be very difficult, both for you and for your doctor, if the local colposcopy clinic simply will not accept your doctor's referral; if you persist, however, your local clinic can usually be persuaded to give you an appointment. And there are clinics which will accept referrals, even from outside their area, although you may have to travel to be seen. Even if you have to wait several months to be seen, at least you will then have been properly investigated. You would, after all, have spent at least that much time having repeat smears.

At the risk of sounding boring and repetitive, we stress again that abnormal cells take *years* to develop into cancer cells, so a few months here and there will not place you at risk.

3

SOME TECHNICAL TERMS

NO ENDOCERVICAL CELLS SEEN. NEGATIVE

22 CYTOLOGY REPORT			Fold

No endocervical cells seen.

23 EVIDENCE OF NEOPLASIA CYTOLOGICAL PATTERN SUGGESTS:	24 INFLAMMATION	25 FURTHER INVESTIGATION SUGGESTED
Inadequate specimen 1	Severe Inflammatory Change 1	Repeat smear in months 1
Negative 2	Trichomonas 2	or after treatment 2
Mild dysplasia 3		Colposcopy 16
Severe dysplasia/ carcinoma-in-situ 4	Candida 4	Cervical biopsy 4
Carcinoma-in-situ/? invasive 5	Viral 8	Uterine curettage 8
? Glandular neoplasia 6	Signature	date
	Fold	

Smear form result: negative.

This is the commonest of the written comments on a smear report. The alternative is 'Endocervical cells seen. Negative'.

Endocervical cells come from the squamo-columnar junction. In Chapter 2 we mentioned that this is an important area, because any changes in the cells are likely to begin

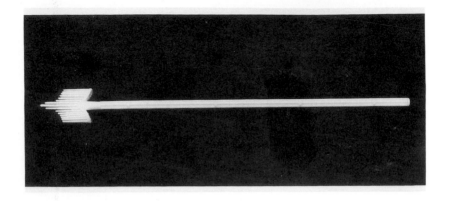

Photograph of Cervex brush.

around there. If there are no endocervical cells present in the smear sample, it means we cannot be sure that this important area is normal. Nevertheless, the rest of the cervix has been checked and contains no abnormality. The smear is therefore negative, but not ideal. For this reason, such smears should be repeated sooner than would usually be recommended for a negative smear – perhaps in six months or a year. The actual timing will depend on the woman's previous smears. For example, if this is her first smear ever, or if the last one was more than two years ago, it would be better to repeat the smear in six months. However, if she has had several completely negative smears at regular intervals of not more than two years, then repeating the smear in a year would be perfectly adequate.

About half the smears which are taken in this country do not show endocervical cells. This is not just due to the incompetence of the people taking them! There are various technical problems in picking up endocervical cells. The most important of these is that the all-important area is often buried deep in the cervical canal, and can be very difficult to reach. This is why new types of spatula and the cytobrush have been developed. These were discussed in Chapter 1 (see page 7). Studies have shown that these new spatulae can improve the pick-up rate of endocervical cells to a level of about 70 per cent, while with a cytobrush a 90 per cent success rate can be achieved.

In addition, the Cervex brush has just become available, which aims to combine the positive features of the cytobrush and the spatulae. An early trial suggests it may be as effective, but further trials are still required to evaluate its potential fully.

Improving the quality of cervical smears in this way also helps to improve the false negative rate; this will be discussed further in Chapter 9.

CERVICAL ECTOPY OR EROSION

Smear form result showing cervical erosion.

This is a harmless condition of the cervix, and is particularly common in women who are pregnant, have had children, or are on the combined oral contraceptive pill.

It simply means that there are many soft columnar cells on the outside surface of the cervix. Normally these cells are hidden in the cervical canal and the outside surface is covered with squamous cells. Columnar cells have a good blood supply, so they look red. In large numbers, they give the cervix a 'grazed' look, which is why the appearance has been described as an erosion. A better description is an ectropion, which is derived from the Greek words meaning eversion (to turn inside-out), as this more accurately describes what has happened.

If you have a large erosion you may notice that you seem to be getting more discharge than in the past. This discharge is the same as the normal non-itchy odourless discharge all women have, but there is more of it. Also, you may get some spotting after intercourse. Columnar cells have a good blood supply (which causes the spotting) and they are also well supplied with glands which produce a normal discharge.

If either of these symptoms become a nuisance, the condition can easily be dealt with by cryotherapy or freezing ('kryos' in Greek means 'frost'). All that happens with this treatment is that a small, very cold metal instrument is held onto the cervix for a couple of minutes; it doesn't hurt, and the treatment is carried out in the outpatient clinic. The only side effect of the treatment is that you get some discharge for a few weeks afterwards (and after all, discharge is what you had before!). If you are having no symptoms (and the majority of women are quite unaware that they have an erosion), there is no need to have any treatment.

CLUE CELLS SUGGESTIVE OF GARDNERELLA

Gardnerella is a bacterium which is very common. It lives in the vagina normally, and usually causes no problems at all. However, if it is there in very large numbers it can cause a slightly smelly discharge, which is not usually itchy. Sometimes

21 CLINICAL DATA (PREVIOUS TREATMENT INCLUDING RADIO THERAPY/CHEMOTHERAPY)			Fold
signature			

22 CYTOLOGY REPORT			Fold

Clue cells suggestive of gardnerella.

23 EVIDENCE OF NEOPLASIA CYTOLOGICAL PATTERN SUGGESTS:	24 INFLAMMATION	25 FURTHER INVESTIGATION SUGGESTED
	Severe Inflammatory Change 1	Repeat smear
Inadequate specimen 1		in months 1
Negative 2	Trichomonas 2	or after treatment 2

Smear form result showing gardnerella.

it can cause a fishy discharge, which is most noticeable after intercourse.

'Clue cells' are just ordinary epithelial (surface lining) cells, to which these bacteria become attached, giving a characteristic appearance under the microscope. They can be seen on a smear slide and, if so, are mentioned by the cytologists just for information. Gardnerella does not cause any kind of cell change which would lead to cervical cancer – they are 'innocent bystanders'.

Should anything be done if gardnerella shows up on your smear? Well, there are almost as many opinions as there are doctors. This is mainly because there is a great debate as to whether in fact these bacteria are 'normal' in the vagina or not. Some doctors think that they are perfectly harmless and that they do not need to be got rid of at all. Others think that they should always be treated if found. And there is the school of compromise which says they should be treated only if the woman is suffering with a discharge.

And as if that was not enough, there is yet another debate as to whether or not they can be passed on during sex. Men certainly don't seem to suffer any symptoms, even if they have the bacteria – but, the question is, can they reinfect their partner, and does it matter if they do? Again, there are two schools of thought; one says that there is no need to treat the man, while the other says men should always be treated.

As you can guess, your treatment will depend on which combination of opinions your doctor holds. There is certainly a trend towards treating women who say they have a discharge. However, this discharge might actually be due to some other infection. The counsel of perfection would therefore be to have a full check-up at a special clinic, which has the facilities to check for all kinds of vaginal infections, whether sexually transmitted or not. It also seems sensible (in our opinion) to treat the partner, just in case the infection keeps being passed back and forth; after all, even a minor infection like candida (thrush or monilia) can be passed on. However, many doctors will merely treat the woman and see if her discharge goes away.

And what is the treatment? It consists of a five-day course of an antibiotic called metronidazole (also called Flagyl). Some people can feel sick while taking these pills, and you should certainly never drink alcohol while on them – unless you are

rid of, and has a tendency to recur. The best treatment for candida is to avoid things that bring it on in the first place. Obviously, antibiotics can be necessary, but perfumed soaps, bubble baths and so on can be avoided. The treatment is usually a course of vaginal pessaries for three nights, together with cream for the outer genital area. Sometimes one stronger pessary is used instead of the three. It is usually a good idea for the male partner to use some cream, though he is unlikely to have any symptoms himself. The idea is mainly to protect you in case he has picked up any spores which will come your way again when you have sex.

Although thrush is a common cause of vaginal discharge and itching, you should not immediately assume this is what you have if you develop such symptoms. Many other infections, such as trichomonas (see below), can cause very similar symptoms, but require different treatment. Ideally, you should be tested in a genito-urinary medicine (special) clinic before any treatment is started. Sometimes you and your doctor may be so sure it is thrush that you will be given treatment without testing. However, if your symptoms do not go away, or recur almost immediately, make sure you are tested for other infections.

TRICHOMONAS (TV)

23 EVIDENCE OF NEOPLASIA CYTOLOGICAL PATTERN SUGGESTS:		24 INFLAMMATION		25 FURTHER INVESTIGATION SUGGESTED	
		Severe Inflammatory Change	1	Repeat smear	
Inadequate specimen	1	Trichomonas	(2)	in months	1
Negative	2			or after treatment	2
Mild dysplasia	3	Candida	4	Colposcopy	16
Severe dysplasia/ carcinoma-in-situ	4	Viral	8	Cervical biopsy	4
Carcinoma-in-situ/? invasive	5			Uterine curettage	8
? Glandular neoplasia	6	Signature		date	

Smear form result showing trichomonas.

30

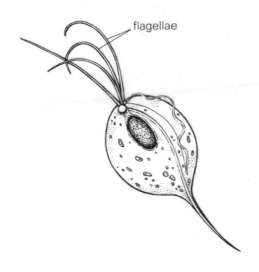

flagellae

Trichomonas vaginalis.

Trichomonas vaginalis is a one-celled organism called a protozoan. (This is derived from the Greek 'proto' meaning 'first' and 'zoion' meaning 'animal', i.e. it is a very primitive life form.) Trichomonas is very interesting to look at under the microscope. It is a pear-shaped organism, which moves around by using its hairs, or flagellae, like oars. In fact, it derives its name from this appearance; 'trichos' means 'hair' in Greek, and 'monas' means 'a unit'. Just to make things more complicated, they then called the hairs 'flagellae' (which means 'whip' in Latin) because of their whip-like motion when the trichomonas swims.

How do creatures that swim get onto your smear? They arrive during sex. Although it is *theoretically* possible to catch trichomonas from swimming pools or lavatory seats, you're kidding yourself if you believe this. Trichomonas in fact is a very common sexually transmitted disease, often causing no symptoms at all in a man. He may therefore be quite unaware he is passing the infection on. Not only may he be unaware he has it, even tests at a sexually transmitted disease clinic often do not show it up in men. You, too, may have been quite unaware of any infection. However, usually, trichomonas in a woman causes a frothy nasty discharge, which smells of old

31

fish and can be very itchy. It may also sometimes cause a little bleeding after intercourse. As with thrush, it may be mistaken for cystitis.

The trouble with trichomonas is that it makes cervical smears very difficult to read, and sometimes it can actually produce an appearance which mimics pre-cancer in the cervical cells. However, it does not cause cancer, and these changes disappear completely after treatment with antibiotics. For this reason, you will be asked to have another smear after your treatment.

The treatment for trichomonas is a five-day course of the antibiotic called metronidazole. This is a useful antibiotic which is also used to treat gardnerella (see above). During the course, you should not drink alcohol, as it will make you feel sick. It is very important that your partner should be treated as well, whether or not he has symptoms, and even if tests show nothing, otherwise you will be reinfected when you have sex with him again.

Once again, it is important to remember that if your symptoms do not clear up after the course of antibiotics, or recur soon afterwards, you should go to a genito-urinary medicine clinic for thorough testing.

ACTINOMYCES FILAMENTS SEEN

Actinomyces is a bacterium which lives normally, and without causing any problems, in the mouth and intestines. However, in women who have an intra-uterine contraceptive device (IUD or coil) fitted it is occasionally found in the vagina, in which case it will show up on the smear. Again it is reported merely for information and *not* because it can cause cells on the cervix to become abnormal.

The trouble with actinomyces is that very, very occasionally it can cause a serious pelvic infection. For this reason it cannot be ignored. Your doctor should check that you are not experiencing any pelvic pain, pain on intercourse, or discharge. If you are, he or she will examine you, and it is likely your IUD will need to be removed and a different form of contraception chosen for the future. Sometimes treatment with penicillin may be needed.

If actinomyces has shown up on the smear but you are not

12 MARITAL STATE	13 PREGNANCIES	14 CONDITION		DATE OF	DAY	MTH	YR
	Total births	Pregnant 1		15 THIS TEST			
Single 1	(live and still)	Post-natal (under 12 weeks) 2					
Married 2		IUCD fitted 16		16 LMP (1st day)			
Widowed/	Total of	On oral contraceptive 4					
Divorced 3	abortions and miscarriages	On other hormones 8 (specify in Box 21)		17 LAST TEST			
				18 NO PREVIOUS TEST (put x)			

19 SYMPTOMS			20 APPEARANCE OF CERVIX
Discharge 1	Post-menopausal bleeding 8		Normal 1
			Eroded 2
Post-coital bleeding 2			Cervicitis 4
	Other symptoms 16		Polyps 8
Inter-menstrual bleeding 4	(Specify in Box 21)		Malignant 16

21 CLINICAL DATA (PREVIOUS TREATMENT INCLUDING RADIO THERAPY/CHEMOTHERAPY) **Fold**

signature

22 CYTOLOGY REPORT **Fold**

Actinomyces filaments seen.

23 EVIDENCE OF NEOPLASIA CYTOLOGICAL PATTERN SUGGESTS:	24 INFLAMMATION	25 FURTHER INVESTIGATION SUGGESTED
Inadequate specimen 1	Severe Inflammatory Change 1	Repeat smear in months 1
Negative 2	Trichomonas 2	or after treatment 2
Mild dysplasia 3		Colposcopy 16
Severe dysplasia/ carcinoma-in-situ 4	Candida 4	Cervical biopsy 4
Carcinoma-in-situ/? invasive 5	Viral 8	Uterine curettage 8
? Glandular neoplasia 6	Signature	date

Smear form results showing actinomyces filaments.

33

having any problems, there are two possible ways of dealing with the situation. One is for your doctor to tell you what to look out for, in terms of pain and discharge, and for you to see your doctor immediately if you are worried. Since this type of serious infection is rare, a 'watch and wait' policy is not unreasonable.

However, it has been shown that in the vast majority of cases the actinomyces can be got rid of just by removing the present IUD and replacing it with a new one. (The new one should be a copper-containing IUD.) A smear should be taken three months later, and then yearly after that. If actinomyces no longer shows up, then all is well. This is a less worrying approach than the 'watch and wait' policy, so it is the one most commonly used.

The older your IUD, the more likely actinomyces is to be present. However, even if your IUD is left in for five years, there is only a 20 per cent chance of actinomyces appearing, and then only a minute risk of a serious infection. You should therefore not be alarmed, but the situation should be dealt with, just in case.

INFLAMMATORY SMEAR

The 'inflammatory' smear is a constant source of argument amongst doctors. For a start, the term can mean different things to different people. Cytologists classify abnormalities in cells mainly by looking at the nucleus of the cell. The grades of abnormality are based on how abnormal the nucleus is, i.e. a mild degree of abnormality becomes mild dysplasia, a severe degree of abnormality becomes severe dysplasia.

If the degree of nuclear abnormality is not enough to be described as CIN 1, then it may be reported as either 'borderline' or 'inflammatory'. Very mild nuclear changes can be caused by infection; almost any type of vaginal infection can be the culprit, even candida (thrush). In addition, 'inflammatory change' can be caused by the wart and herpes viruses. If the cytologist finds an infection he can recognise from the smear, he will mark it in section 24 on the form.

Unfortunately, not all infections show up on a smear, nor are all 'inflammatory' smears caused by infection. The problem is that the assessment of nuclear abnormality is to

23 EVIDENCE OF NEOPLASIA CYTOLOGICAL PATTERN SUGGESTS:	24 INFLAMMATION	25 FURTHER INVESTIGATION SUGGESTED
Inadequate specimen 1	Severe Inflammatory Change ①	Repeat smear in months 1
Negative 2	Trichomonas 2	or after treatment 2
Mild dysplasia 3	Candida 4	Colposcopy 16
Severe dysplasia/ carcinoma-in-situ 4	Viral 8	Cervical biopsy 4
Carcinoma-in-situ/? invasive 5		Uterine curettage 8
? Glandular neoplasia 6	Signature	date
	Fold	

23 EVIDENCE OF NEOPLASIA CYTOLOGICAL PATTERN SUGGESTS:	24 INFLAMMATION	25 FURTHER INVESTIGATION SUGGESTED
Inadequate specimen 1	~~Severe~~ Inflammatory Change ①	Repeat smear in months 1
Negative 2	Trichomonas 2	or after treatment 2
Mild dysplasia 3	Candida 4	Colposcopy 16
Severe dysplasia/ carcinoma-in-situ 4	Viral 8	Cervical biopsy 4
Carcinoma-in-situ/? invasive 5		Uterine curettage 8
? Glandular neoplasia 6	Signature	date
	Fold	

Smear form results showing both severe inflammatory change and inflammatory change.

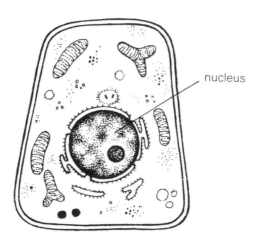

nucleus

Diagram of a cell. The nucleus is responsible for directing any process of change which goes on inside a cell.

some extent subjective; that is, it depends on who looks at it. One cytologist may decide to report a smear as inflammatory, while another would report the very same smear as mild dysplasia. Indeed, it has been shown that up to one in four persistent (i.e. repeatedly) 'inflammatory' smears do, in fact, have some degree of dysplasia, or even cancer. At present, an 'inflammatory' smear is often ignored. After all, it has been reported as negative, so why do anything about it? Some doctors do not themselves understand what an 'inflammatory' smear means.

Take the case of Jane, a happily married 34-year-old part-time secretary. She had two children, Sarah aged ten and Vicky aged six. She was always careful to attend for her smears, which her GP had been doing for her since her first pregnancy. Jane's first smear was normal, but her second, four years later, showed severe inflammatory change. Jane was pregnant with Vicky at the time, had an itchy vaginal discharge and was treated with pessaries and cream for thrush. She was unaware of the result of her smear, believing it to be completely normal. After Vicky's birth she was very busy, with a baby and a toddler in the house, and forgot to attend for her post-natal check – in any case, she was well and had been through it before.

Five years went by, and she received a reminder to attend for a routine smear. She was glad, because she had been meaning to go to her GP anyway. During the last few months she had noticed a little spotting of blood after making love with her husband. It did not happen every time, but she wanted to ask what it could be.

Her GP looked concerned when she told him. He examined her and took a smear. Two weeks later she received a letter asking her to attend the surgery. She was told that she had an abnormal smear and would be seen a week later in the colposcopy clinic at the local hospital. There Jane learnt that she had the beginnings of cervical cancer. She was advised to have a hysterectomy. Luckily, the cancer had not spread and she needed no more treatment after that. Today she is alive and well.

Jane was lucky. There have been unfortunate women who repeatedly had smears showing severe inflammatory change and who were found to have invasive cancer when they were finally seen at a colposcopy clinic.

There is a possible third reason for a smear to be inflammatory. If a woman has stopped having periods (i.e. has been through the menopause), her body stops producing the hormone oestrogen. This lack of oestrogen may make her vagina dry and the skin lining it thin or atrophic ('trophe' in Greek means 'nourishment', while the prefix 'a' means 'without'). Sometimes atrophic cells can show changes which are indistinguishable from inflammatory ones.

So, what should be done about an 'inflammatory' smear? First of all, you must find out about it – you are very likely not to be informed, or told that you have a negative smear. You may need to ask specifically 'Was there any inflammation shown on my smear?'

And remember that the majority of inflammatory smears will not be due to dysplasia. It is much more likely that there is, in fact, some form of infection. The best place to be checked for any kind of vaginal infection is a genito-urinary medicine clinic (also called a sexually transmitted disease clinic or a special clinic). This type of clinic has facilities for checking a wide variety of vaginal infections (whether sexually transmitted or not), and can often give you the majority of results immediately. Neither GPs nor family planning clinics have such a wide range of tests available, and they have to wait about a week for results to come through.

Once you (and, of course, your partner) have been checked and treated for any infection, you should have another smear in about three to six months' time. If this shows any abnormality, or is again 'inflammatory', you should be referred for colposcopy. Even if the repeat smear is negative, you should make sure you have another smear in about 18 months' time, to be on the safe side.

If it is likely that the smear may be showing atrophic cells, a six-week course of a vaginal oestrogen cream can be tried, followed by a repeat smear. Again, if the second smear is abnormal, you should be referred for colposcopy.

4

THE COLPOSCOPY EXAMINATION

PRELIMINARIES

A colposcopy clinic is an outpatient clinic, much like any other, so bring a good book or some magazines, as you are bound to be kept waiting. This does not mean, however, that you should aim to arrive late; there is a law somewhere which states that if you arrive late for your appointment, the clinic will, for once, be running on time.

A gown will probably be provided for you, but you are unlikely to have to remove many clothes. However, bear in mind that a tight skirt will be a disadvantage when you are lying on a couch with your legs in stirrups. Trousers may seem sensible, but, of course, will have to be taken off; in many ways a loose wide skirt is the best idea.

Many women find it reassuring to bring someone with them. It can be very frightening to be in a strange place, awaiting an internal examination on your own. A partner, friend or relative can make a great deal of difference. It means you have someone to share the long wait with, and to give you moral support once you are actually having the examination.

Don't be afraid to ask questions once you are with the doctor. Clinics are always busy, and women often feel that they will be taking up 'too much of the doctor's valuable time'. In fact, that time is meant to be spent looking after *you*. Making sure that you understand what is happening to you is part of the reason for your appointment, and who better to explain it to you than the expert doing the colposcopy?

You are bound to be asked some questions, relating to your periods, the type of contraception you use, any operations or illnesses you may have had in the past, whether you smoke, and so on. One question you are guaranteed to be asked is the first day of your last period. You have no idea how irritating it is to watch the twentieth woman of the morning scrambling around in her handbag for her diary, and then to spend the next five minutes waiting while she tries to work it out – the time could be so much better spent answering your questions. Remembering when your last period started is something you can do while you are sitting, bored, in the waiting room; it will be worth it just to see the doctor's face light up with a grateful smile.

THE EXAMINATION

Once both the doctor's and your questions have been answered, you will be asked to lie down on the colposcopy couch. As you can see, it is slightly different from a normal

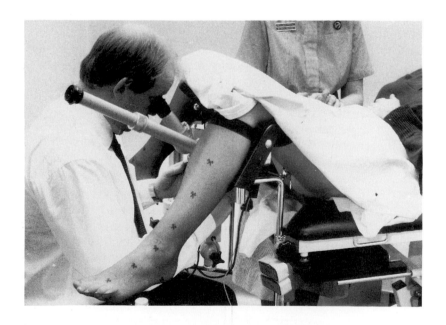

Using the colposcope.

40

couch; it is angled, the bottom end is missing and stirrups or leg rests are attached. The angling and the stirrups are necessary for achieving the best possible view of your cervix. (The womb is actually quite mobile, and changes its angle according to your position.)

Some clinics have pictures on the ceiling to keep you occupied, while others may have a video set up so you can actually watch the examination yourself (although if this does not appeal, you are quite at liberty to ask for it to be switched off).

There will probably be some fumbling around while the colposcope is moved into position. The colposcope looks pretty alarming, with knobs and switches and arms all over the place, but in fact it's just a large magnifying glass with a light source attached.

The next thing that happens is that a speculum is inserted gently into your vagina. This is exactly the same procedure as for a smear, and sometimes the doctor does in fact take a smear. The main difference is that, unlike a smear test, the speculum has to stay inside you until the examination is over (about five minutes). Remember that, as with a smear, it will only be uncomfortable if you are tense. Breathing slowly and deeply in and out may help you relax.

Your cervix will then be wiped with some cotton wool soaked in acetic acid, which is just dilute vinegar; it does not sting, but it may feel a little cold. The acetic acid stains abnormal areas on the cervix white, and the degree of whiteness gives some idea of the degree of abnormality. It takes a little time for the white areas to show up, so at this point you will probably find yourself discussing the weather with the doctor and nurse.

Sometimes, iodine is also wiped onto the cervix, which can cause a slight burning sensation. Iodine is good at showing up the abnormal areas; it is easier to see than the white stains that might be produced by the acetic acid, and so makes taking a biopsy easier (see below). If iodine is used, you will get a dark brown discharge for a day or two afterwards, because of its colour.

If there is an abnormal area on your cervix, a tiny biopsy will be taken from it. This is a piece of tissue about the size of a pin-head; some women feel a short sharp pain, but you may be quite unaware that it has been done. However, you are likely to have a mild period pain for a short while afterwards. Taking the biopsy may cause a little bleeding, so a tampon will probably be put in before the speculum is removed. And then it's all over.

A biopsy specimen is much more accurate than a smear in deciding the actual grade of abnormality. Instead of loose cells, there is a very small, but solid, piece of tissue which can be looked at in detail, piece by piece, under a microscope. Because it is all in one piece, not only can the abnormal area be graded, but it is possible to tell how deeply it extends. Obviously, these things are all important in deciding how much treatment you will need.

Biopsy specimens are placed in a preservative solution and sent to a special laboratory to be looked at. This means they join a queue and, of course, the actual procedure takes time, so the results will not normally be available for a week or two, except for urgent cases, when the results can be obtained within 48 hours. This is a shame because it means that you cannot have an answer at the time of your colposcopy. However, the doctor doing the colposcopy may be able to give you at least an idea of what your treatment is likely to be.

Once it is all over you will be told how long you are likely to wait for an appointment for treatment, if this is necessary. Again, this will vary depending on where you live, on the degree of abnormality which the biopsy shows and, to some extent, on what is available at that hospital. There are several different forms of treatment, which we shall look at in the next chapter.

UNSATISFACTORY COLPOSCOPY

There is a situation in which a colposcopy is considered technically unsatisfactory. This happens when the area of abnormality extends deep into the cervical canal and the doctor cannot see where it ends. Obviously, if you can't see it you don't know what's going on; there is always the danger that the bit you can't see is actually worse than the part which is visible. Because of this, the only way to be absolutely safe is to perform a cone biopsy. This is described towards the end of the next chapter. It is not done at the time of your visit to the colposcopy clinic, so you will be given a separate appointment.

It does not mean there is anything seriously wrong – it is just that the colposcopy did not provide a complete view. The vast majority of colposcopies though are perfectly satisfactory.

5

TREATING A CERVICAL ABNORMALITY

This chapter deals with the treatment of pre-cancerous cervical abnormalities; the treatment of cancer itself is described briefly in the next chapter. There are a number of different ways of treating pre-cancerous lesions, as they are called, and to a great extent the actual choice depends on the preference of the individual gynaecologist and which methods are actually available in his or her department.

The general principle behind all these forms of treatment is the same; namely, to destroy all the abnormal cells with the minimum disruption to normal tissue. We shall discuss their relative advantages and disadvantages as we go along.

As a general rule, most gynaecologists prefer not to perform treatment during the heavy days of a period. The blood tends to obscure the field of view, making the procedure technically more difficult. Moreover, bleeding due to the treatment is more likely because the area is already 'primed' for bleeding. If you have a period on the day of your treatment it is a good idea to ring up and check whether you should actually come in or not. You should also inform the doctor if you have become pregnant in the interval between your colposcopy and treatment appointments. Pregnancy can alter the way in which you will be monitored and treated; this will be discussed towards the end of the chapter.

No matter what type of treatment you receive, it is very important that you attend for follow-up appointments. You will normally be seen twice in the first year after treatment. At each visit a colposcopy will be performed and a smear may be taken. If any areas of abnormality show up again, a biopsy will be taken and you may need to have further treatment. This only happens in 5–10 per cent of cases, but obviously it is important that those women are not missed. And once you have been discharged from the colposcopy clinic, remember that you must continue to have yearly smears.

There are four types of treatment available – cryotherapy, electrodiathermy, cold coagulation and laser treatment. The prerequisites for their use are that the *whole* area of abnormality can be seen through the colposcope, and that there is no suggestion of an actual cancer being present. If either of these criteria are not fulfilled, cone biopsy has to be performed; this will be described towards the end of this chapter.

The first step in any treatment is a colposcopy, so that the abnormal areas can be mapped out, usually using iodine.

CRYOTHERAPY

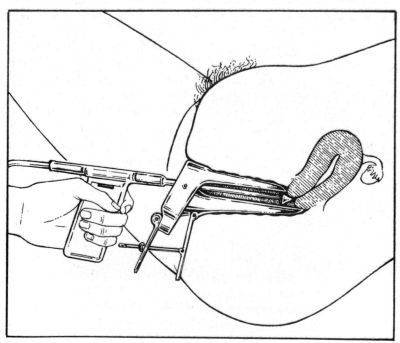

Applying the cryoprobe to the cervix.

This method destroys the abnormal cells by freezing ('kryos' means 'frost' in Greek). As you can see, the tip of the cryoprobe fits onto the cervix. It is attached to a pressurised supply of carbon dioxide or nitrous oxide, which becomes very cold when the pressure is suddenly released and allowed to reach the tip of the probe. In fact, the tip actually becomes covered with frost during the treatment.

The cryoprobe is usually held onto the cervix for about three minutes at first. The area is then allowed to thaw for about five minutes before refreezing for another three minutes. This is usually sufficient to destroy the affected cells, but if the abnormal cell area is large two treatments may be needed. This method is also used in the treatment of cervical erosions (see Chapter 3). For that purpose only one freezing application, lasting three minutes, is needed.

Cryotherapy is a simple technique which is performed in the outpatient clinic without any anaesthetic. During the procedure you may experience a type of mild period pain, and some women do feel a little faint afterwards. Painkillers are often provided, and it is certainly a good idea to have someone with you who can accompany you home if necessary. Afterwards you will have a watery discharge, which is often quite heavy for about three weeks and then gradually diminishes. It is usually gone by six weeks.

Cryotherapy is most successful in the treatment of mild abnormalities, such as CIN 1 or 2. However it is not always as good for treating CIN 3 because it is difficult to get deep enough to be absolutely sure there are no abnormal cells left. In addition, it can result in a certain amount of scarring on the cervix, which can make follow-up more difficult. Its advantages, certainly in the treatment of mild abnormalities, are that it is simple, requires no anaesthesia, takes only a short time and is cheap.

ELECTRODIATHERMY

This method relies on high temperatures (about 1,000 °C) to destroy the abnormal cells. The heat is applied through an electrode which is placed on the cervix. Unfortunately this is a painful procedure, so it has to be performed under a general anaesthetic.

The heat is applied until no more mucus is seen coming from the cervical glands. It is important these gland crypts should be destroyed because abnormal cells can extend downwards to that depth. Once there are no gland cells, indicated by the lack of mucus, it is very unlikely any abnormal cells are left.

You can expect a blood-stained discharge for three to four weeks after treatment, but the cervix usually heals well, with little or no scarring. This method is very successful in treating all degrees of CIN. However its major disadvantage is that it has to be performed under general anaesthetic.

Nowadays a short procedure like this is usually done as a day case. You come into hospital having not eaten or drunk for at least six hours, the treatment is performed shortly after your arrival, and you go home on the same day. Although having a general anaesthetic means you will be unconscious, the type used is very mild, so you wake up rapidly afterwards. Some women do feel a little sick and drowsy afterwards, so you are normally advised to arrange for someone to come and collect you, preferably by car. However, you can expect to feel quite well, often by the same evening and certainly by the next day.

COLD COAGULATION

The cold coagulator also relies on heat to destroy abnormal cells. It is called 'cold' because the amount of heat used is only about a tenth of that in electrodiathermy. Once again, the heat is generated by an electric current which heats up the metal of the probes. The treatment only lasts a minute or two, and does not require an anaesthetic. As in cryotherapy, you may experience a mild period-type pain, and painkillers are often given to help this. Following treatment, as after electrodiathermy, you are likely to have a blood-stained discharge for up to about four weeks. The cervix heals well, though, with little or no scarring.

This method has the advantage of not requiring an anaesthetic, and is very successful at treating CIN 1 and 2 lesions. It can also be used for some CIN 3 lesions but, again, there can be difficulty in achieving the required depth.

LASER TREATMENT

The word laser is actually derived from light amplification by stimulated emission of radiation, so you can see why they shortened it. A laser works by producing an extremely powerful and concentrated fine beam of light energy. This beam can then be focused accurately by using mirrors and lenses. Because it is such a fine beam, it can be used very accurately, not just to destroy tissue, but also for cutting. The laser destroys tissue by vapourisation; the cells are heated so rapidly they simply evaporate. It is attached to a colposcope, so the area to be treated can be accurately mapped out and watched throughout the procedure.

Laser treatment is usually performed under local anaesthetic; you are given a couple of anaesthetic injections actually into the cervix. This is very similar to having an anaesthetic injection at the dentist, but is less painful, and the majority of women are quite unaware it has been done. The procedure is usually carried out in the colposcopy clinic, and you sit on a normal colposcopy couch. The laser machine itself looks like a large box attached to the colposcope. You may be aware of a hissing noise; this is merely a suction machine which clears the field of view for the doctor, and removes any unpleasant odour due to the vapourisation.

Sometimes the doctors and nurses wear protective glasses during the treatment. This is because there is always the danger of the beam being reflected, for example off the shiny surfaces of the speculum. You are at the safe end from this point of view; the most likely person to suffer is the doctor performing the treatment, as it could be reflected back into his or her face. Luckily, the chances of this happening are very small indeed.

Laser treatment takes about ten minutes, and you may feel a slight period-type pain during this time. If you feel any other pain, tell the doctor; stopping for a moment, or moving the beam on to another area will get rid of it almost straight away. Do your best not to move suddenly during the treatment as, obviously, this will move your anatomy in relation to the beam. At the end of the treatment, antiseptic cream is usually applied to the cervix to help prevent any infection.

Some women do feel shaky afterwards, mainly because of their anxiety and the thought of what is happening to them. It

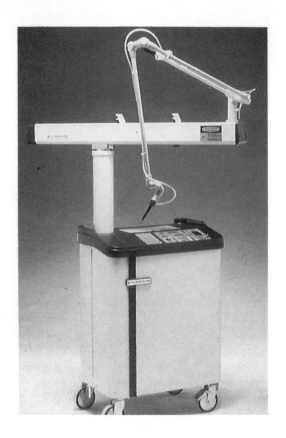

Laser machine.

is therefore often helpful for your partner to come along and literally hold your hand during the procedure. It is certainly a good idea for someone to be present who can accompany you home. Occasionally, if a women is very anxious, or if extensive treatment is needed, laser treatment is performed under a general anaesthetic. However, this is very much the exception rather than the rule.

The cervix heals extremely well after laser treatment, but you will notice some bleeding for up to two weeks afterwards. This may sometimes be as heavy as a period. Persistent bleeding worries many women, and departments where laser treatment is performed are used to women phoning up for advice, which will be readily given. Very occasionally they may ask you to come in so they can have a look; in practice it is rare for the bleeding to need any extra treatment, but it is reassuring for both you and them.

A laser machine is a very expensive item, but this form of treatment has a number of advantages. It can be used to treat any degree of CIN, as the depth of treatment can be easily and precisely controlled. It does not usually require a general anaesthetic. Healing takes place very rapidly and there is no residual scarring. Another important advantage is that the cervix is remoulded during the treatment so that the endocervical canal does not become too tight. This means that follow-up is much easier as the crucial area is easily visible. In addition, it is now beginning to replace surgery as a method of performing cone biopsies (see below).

AFTER TREATMENT

Whatever method has been used, the cervix must be given time to heal. During this time it is particularly vulnerable to infection, as well as to mechanical damage. For this reason you will be asked not to have sexual intercourse for at least three weeks (possibly up to six weeks), and even then it is advisable for your partner to use a sheath for another three weeks. Similarly, you should not use tampons or douches during that time. By three months your cervix will be completely healed, and, particularly following laser treatment, nobody, not even a gynaecologist, will be able to tell that you've had any treatment.

Some clinics ask to see you again after three months, just to check that everything has healed satisfactorily, and you should certainly be seen at six and twelve months after treatment for a colposcopy and a smear, to make sure the abnormal cells have all disappeared. It is important you do not miss these checks, as none of the methods guarantee a 100-per-cent cure straight away. Some women need two treatments before they are completely clear. However, the success rate after one treatment is usually 90–5 per cent.

These treatments for cervical pre-cancer will have no effect on your future fertility, nor will you be at any greater risk of having a miscarriage afterwards. In fact, it has been observed that women actually seem to be more likely to become pregnant shortly after laser treatment.

51

AN ABNORMAL SMEAR IN PREGNANCY

In general, nobody is keen to treat the cervix during pregnancy. There is always the possibility of bringing on a miscarriage, bleeding tends to be much worse and more difficult to stop, and the whole thing makes the woman very anxious. Luckily, in the majority of cases it is not necessary to do anything at all until after the baby has been safely delivered; nine months is, after all, not a very long time, and pre-cancer takes considerably longer than that to become cancer.

However, it is known that pre-cancers, like genital warts, tend to progress faster during pregnancy. Pregnancy is a time when immunity is relatively low, partly to avoid rejection of the baby by the mother's body (this does mean, though, that infections can thrive). For this reason, you will be kept under close surveillance throughout and immediately after the pregnancy. You will probably be seen in the colposcopy clinic at about three-monthly intervals, and then a couple of months after delivery. At each visit you will be carefully assessed to make sure there is no sign of cancer, and a smear will be taken. Biopsies are usually avoided during pregnancy, mainly because of bleeding problems. Apart from these checks, though, cervical pre-cancer should not make any other difference to your pregnancy or your delivery.

Difficulties do arise if early cancer does develop during pregnancy. Many factors have to be taken into account, including the degree of cancer and how far pregnant the woman is; it is impossible to give general guidelines, as each case has to be assessed individually. Your gynaecologist will discuss all the options with you, and your feelings about what you want to do will determine the final decision as to your treatment and the pregnancy.

CONE BIOPSY

Cone biopsy is the removal of a cone-shaped area of the cervix. Before the advent of colposcopy, this was the only treatment available for an abnormal smear, but nowadays it only needs to be performed under three circumstances.

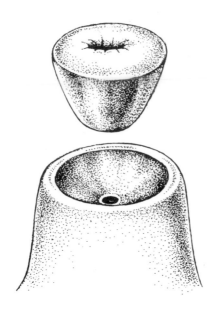

Cone biopsy.

1   If the area of abnormality extends so far up into the
    cervical canal that its upper limit cannot be seen through
    the colposcope. There is then the danger of missing a more
    serious abnormality than that which can be seen.
2   If the woman's smears are consistently and persistently
    abnormal, even though nothing can be seen to account for
    them on colposcopy. Again, there is the danger of missing
    an abnormality which cannot be seen through the colpo-
    scope.
3   If, on colposcopy, the doctor is worried that the abnormal
    area may be beginning to turn into a cancer. In this case it
    is important to remove a larger piece of tissue for very
    accurate histology (microscopic examination). In addition,
    a cone biopsy may actually remove the whole abnormality,
    and may then be the only treatment required, even if a
    very early cancer had been diagnosed. In some ways the
    name 'cone biopsy' is misleading, because it both diagno-
    ses and treats the abnormality at the same time.

In practice, about 10 to 15 per cent of all the women
attending a colposcopy clinic have a cone biopsy.

There are now two possible ways of performing a cone biopsy, either surgically or using the laser.

Surgical cone biopsy

If the cone biopsy is to be done surgically you will need to come into hospital for a few days. If your period starts on or just before the day you are supposed to come in, check with the department that this is all right; some gynaecologists prefer not to operate during a period, as this makes bleeding more likely.

This type of operation has to be performed under a light general anaesthetic, so you will be unconscious during it. It only takes about 20 minutes, but you will be asleep for a short time afterwards as well. You normally come into hospital a day before the operation, and stay for a couple of days afterwards. You will not be allowed to eat or drink for at least six hours prior to the anaesthetic and, as with any general anaesthetic, you may feel sick for a few hours afterwards. You are also likely to experience crampy, period-type pain for up to 24 hours afterwards, and you will be given painkillers to help this.

Bleeding for several days after the operation is quite normal. However, sometimes the bleeding can become heavy a few days after you have left hospital. If this happens you should ring the department; they may have to help your body stop the bleeding, usually just by applying pressure to the cervix.

Surgical cone biopsy can lead to a couple of problems. Firstly, the external cervical os (opening) may become very tight afterwards, which can result in painful periods. In contrast, the internal cervical os may become too slack. This depends on how much of the cervix was removed during the cone biopsy. As you can see from the diagrams opposite, it is the length, rather than the width of the cone removed which is important here. Unfortunately, it is not always possible to remove only a short cone; it depends on how far up the cervix the area of abnormality extends.

Damage to the muscle of the internal cervical os can cause problems in pregnancy. The internal os is responsible for keeping the baby in the womb until the beginning of labour; if it becomes weak, there may come a time during pregnancy when the weight of the baby overcomes it and a miscarriage

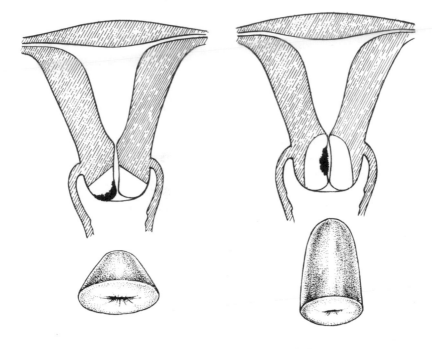

a. 'Short' cone biopsy.   b. 'Long' cone biopsy.

occurs. This often happens after the twelfth week of pregnancy, in contrast to most miscarriages, which happen before then. In order to avoid this problem, a stitch, rather like a purse-string, can be inserted into the cervix during early pregnancy. This stitch is often called a Shirodkar suture, after the doctor who first used it. It is removed once the woman has reached 38 weeks, and she then goes into labour normally.

Damage to the internal os was more common in the days before colposcopy was available. Nowadays, using the colposcope, the area to be removed can be much more accurately mapped out, which means that the doctor does not need to leave such a wide safety margin. This has reduced the size of cone biopsies, and consequently reduced the complications.

Fertility itself (i.e. how likely you are to fall pregnant in the first place) is very rarely reduced by cone biopsy.

Laser cone biopsy

As we mentioned before, the laser can be used as a very powerful, very accurate 'knife'. In many ways it is therefore ideal for use in cone biopsy; it provides not only greater accuracy than a surgical knife, but also leaves virtually no scarring, which means that the complications mentioned above are far less likely to occur.

At present, most laser cone biopsies are done under general anaesthetic. However, in some cases they can be done under local anaesthetic, in a similar manner to ordinary laser treatment. This is obviously an advantage as it means the procedure can be done in the outpatient clinic. In addition, bleeding is less of a problem after a laser cone biopsy, so the woman can often go home on the same day. The other advantage of using the laser is that, as with ordinary laser treatment, the cervix can be remoulded, making the external os less likely to tighten up and therefore improving accessibility during follow-up.

What happens after a cone biopsy?

Unfortunately, the results of the microscopic examination of the tissue removed during the cone biopsy will not be available before you go home. You will therefore probably be given an appointment to come back and discuss them with your doctor about two weeks later.

In the majority of cases, the news will be good. You will be told that the whole area of abnormality was removed and that there was no sign of actual cancer. Remember that many cone biopsies are done purely because of incomplete visibility during the colposcopy, not because there was any suspicion of cancer. In this case you will be followed up in the same way as any other woman who has had treatment for pre-cancer. You will be seen in the colposcopy clinic at roughly six-monthly intervals for the first year, and then often simply advised to have yearly smears.

In some cases, although there is no suggestion of cancer, the area of abnormality may not have been completely removed. We walk a tightrope nowadays, between trying to remove as little of the cervix as possible in order to minimise later complications, and yet remove the entire abnormal area. This is successful most of the time, although it does unfortunately mean that a woman occasionally has to have extra local treatment (e.g. laser treatment) or a second cone biopsy.

The most important feature of the microscopic examination is to show whether or not there has been any spread of abnormal cells through the basement membrane (described in Chapter 1). If this is apparent it is a sign of cancer. However, the degree to which this penetration has occurred is also very important. If there is only very slight spread, the cancer is described as microinvasive. If it has been completely removed by the cone biopsy, no further treatment may be needed. However, if there has been deep and extensive spread through the basement membrane, the cancer is more worrying. Both of these types of cancer are discussed more fully in the next chapter.

HYSTERECTOMY FOR PRE-CANCER OF THE CERVIX

Hysterectomy (removal of the uterus, or womb) is occasionally recommended for pre-cancer if there is already some other reason for having a hysterectomy anyway. For example, if a woman has completed her family, and is having very heavy, painful periods, she may already be thinking of a hysterectomy for this reason. It would then be silly to treat her cervix, only for her to have the whole uterus removed a short time later.

Hysterectomy is, of course, a bigger operation than cone biopsy, involving a week or more in hospital, and several more weeks recovering fully at home. You should make sure you have fully discussed this with your gynaecologist before you reach any final decision.

Hysterectomy for cervical cancer is often performed in a different way to that for pre-cancer, and this will be discussed in the next chapter.

6

CERVICAL CANCER

Up till now all the conditions we have described have been pre-cancers, i.e. although there are abnormal cells present, they have not yet become cancer cells. A detailed account of the treatment of cervical cancer is outside the scope of this book; this chapter is intended only to give an outline of the various possibilities. If you should be unfortunate enough to find that you have cervical cancer, it is important that the person you turn to for information is your gynaecologist. Every woman's case is different, both in the degree of cancer present and her own personal circumstances, and information obtained from books, articles and friends may be very misleading when applied, without expert knowledge, to your own particular case.

CAN I TELL IF I HAVE CERVICAL CANCER?

Probably not. Warning signs may be unusual bleeding – after intercourse, between periods, after the menopause (change of life). In addition, vaginal discharge may occur. However there are other, perfectly innocent, causes of all these symptoms; for example, the commonest cause of vaginal discharge is infection, while the most likely cause of bleeding after intercourse is a cervical erosion (see Chapter 3). Bleeding between periods often occurs in women who are fitted with an intra-uterine contraceptive device (IUD), while bleeding after the menopause may be a sign of hormone deficiency. Nevertheless, if you experience any of these symptoms, you should tell your doctor.

Women who are on the combined pill may sometimes experience bleeding outside their pill-free week. This is not the same as bleeding between periods; it is known as 'break-through bleeding' and may be caused by forgetting a pill, taking antibiotics, having a stomach upset, or simply taking a brand which is not quite right for you. A change to a different brand may solve the problem, so you should mention this to your doctor.

Many early cancers in fact have no symptoms at all, so there is no point waiting until you notice something is wrong. Cervical screening is intended to pick up abnormalities which have no symptoms and which have not yet become cancerous. Only in this way can cervical cancer be prevented.

THE STAGES, OR DEGREES, OF CANCER OF THE CERVIX

Over the years doctors have developed a way of describing the degrees of severity of cervical cancer. This is useful for several reasons. It means that the results of different treatments can be realistically compared. It also means that some predictions can be made of what is likely to happen (for example the chances of cure) if a woman is treated at any given stage.

There are four stages, and each is subdivided into two parts, called a and b. It would be pointless to explain each of these in depth – the definitions are lengthy and require a detailed knowledge of anatomy to understand them. Broadly speaking, they describe how far the cancerous cells have spread. Stage 1 cancer involves only the womb itself. Stage 2 cancer has spread a little way outside the womb, for example into the vagina. In stage 3 it has spread further, but is still within the pelvis. Stage 4 means the cancerous cells have spread outside the pelvis, to the bladder, bowel or even more distant organs like the lungs and liver.

How do cancer cells spread? At first, they just increase in number locally, so that normal cells are pushed aside or squashed. This is called microinvasion. At this point, it is still possible to remove them all just by removing the part of the cervix which is involved. This can be done by cone biopsy, which was described in the previous chapter.

If the cancer cells manage to increase sufficiently in number, they will spread deep enough to reach the lymph channels. Lymph is a liquid which carries white blood cells around the body. These cells are designed to fight any 'intruders', such as bacteria and viruses, and they also attack cancer cells, although not always with success. Unfortunately, the cancer cells can also use the network of lymph channels (which is comparable to the blood-vessel system) to spread to other areas of the body. Once they start to spread the cancer cells will tend to get trapped in the lymph nodes, which are places where the white blood cells congregate in large numbers. (You can think of lymph nodes as being rather like police stations, containing a large number of policemen within a small area, while the roaming white cells in the lymph channels are rather like police patrol cars spread around the city.)

Lymph nodes which have trapped large numbers of cancer cells tend to increase in size, and sometimes become tender. This is why doctors examine the lymph nodes very carefully; it is not possible to see cancer cells moving, but an enlarged lymph node is a marker of spread.

Cervical cancer cells can thus spread from lymph node to lymph node via the lymphatic channels, all the lymph nodes in the body being connected to each other via these channels, just like a network of roads connecting cities and towns. Gradually the cancer cells reach lymph nodes which are further and further away from their original site, which is how they reach organs as far away as the lung. Obviously, the more areas of the body are involved, the more difficult it is to get rid of the cancer. This is the reason why, before any treatment is contemplated, an assessment has to be made of how far the cancer cells are likely to have spread; there is no point in only treating the pelvis if the cancer has already reached the lungs. And this assessment is made more difficult by the fact that not all cancers behave in the same predictable fashion. Some are more aggressive than others – they tend to fight their way into the lymph channels more quickly – and therefore can spread to other parts of the body more rapidly. Unfortunately, it seems that the younger the woman, the more aggressive her cancer is likely to be.

MICROINVASION

This is the name given to the very earliest stage of cancer, called 1a. In fact, there is considerable argument within the medical profession as to exactly what the definition of microinvasion should be, and even whether it is likely to behave like an invasive cancer at all.

If a cancer is described as microinvasive, it means that it has spread literally only a few millimetres through the basement membrane (see Chapter 1). In theory, therefore, it should not yet have reached any lymphatic channels. The problem is, how to prove that it has not reached any lymphatic channels. This is very difficult, and is the reason why a cone biopsy has to be looked at so closely under the microscope. If the specialists are sure that no lymph channels are involved, and the entire area of cancer cells has been removed by the cone biopsy, it should be safe for the woman to have no further treatment – she is cured.

Unfortunately, it is not always possible to be absolutely sure. This is where the personal circumstances of the woman are important in influencing her treatment. For example, if

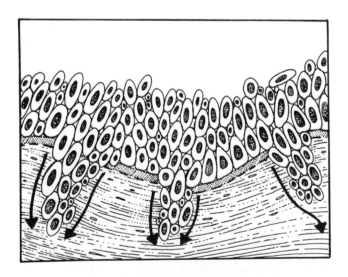

Abnormal cells crossing the basement membrane to the connective tissue.

she has already completed her family, and perhaps has other gynaecological problems, such as heavy periods, then she would be best advised to have a hysterectomy. However, she may be young, single and with no children, and is justifiably likely to be very distressed at the thought of a hysterectomy. In this case, the gynaecologist will explain the problem to her and let her make the final decision. If she only has a cone biopsy, the risk of the cancer spreading cannot be ruled out, although it is likely to be very, very small. With close monitoring in the colposcopy clinic, she may well be prepared to take that risk in order to give herself the opportunity of having a family.

INVASIVE CANCER

By the time a cancer has become obviously invasive, a woman is likely to have symptoms, as described at the beginning of this chapter. A diagnostic cone biopsy will show that the tumour has already spread to the lymph channels. Before any further treatment can be given, however, it is important to find out just how far the cancer has spread.

Various tests will be performed. One of them is likely to be a special X-ray of the kidneys and bladder, called an intravenous pyelogram or urogram (IVP or IVU). This makes use of a special dye which shows up on an X-ray picture. The dye is injected into the woman's arm, travels rapidly in the bloodstream to the kidneys, and X-ray pictures are taken while it is passing through the kidneys and bladder. By comparing the appearance with what is known to be normal, doctors can tell if there is any tumour in these organs.

A chest X-ray will also be taken, to check that there is no cancer in the lungs. Sometimes a special scan is carried out which can show up the lymph nodes in the body. This can help in seeing which ones have been invaded by tumours. There are various other types of scan which can be performed; which ones are chosen will depend partly on what is available at your hospital, and partly on which ones your doctors feel to be most useful in your particular case.

Sometimes your gynaecologist may want to examine the vagina and pelvis under a general anaesthestic, during which he can also examine the bladder directly, using a flexible tube with a built-in light (this is called cystoscopy).

The two main types of treatment used for cervical cancer are surgery and radiotherapy; sometimes only one is used, sometimes they are combined. Chemotherapy is also occasionally used, but usually in those cases where other treatment has not succeeded as well as was hoped. Every woman's case is different, and the treatment will be tailored to her needs. Her age and personal circumstances will always be taken into account, to try and give her the maximum quality, as well as quantity, of life.

SURGICAL TREATMENT

Surgical treatment involves a special type of hysterectomy, often called a Wertheim's or Meig's hysterectomy after the surgeons who developed it. It is a somewhat bigger operation than an ordinary hysterectomy, because the pelvic lymph nodes are removed as well as the uterus. Removing the lymph nodes serves two purposes: firstly, the idea is to remove any tissue which could contain tumour cells; and secondly, by examining the lymph nodes under a microscope, it is possible to tell exactly how far the tumour has in fact spread. In this way, the woman can be given an indication of how successful her treatment is likely to be. The ovaries are not removed unless the woman has gone through the menopause (change of life), in which case they are no longer of any use to her. Hormone replacement therapy can be started soon after she has had the operation.

A Wertheim's hysterectomy is a long operation, lasting several hours. This is partly because of the time required to remove each lymph node, but also because the surgeon has to operate slowly and meticulously to avoid damaging the bladder and the ureters (these are the tubes leading from the bladder down to the outside opening, the urethra, through which you pass urine).

When you wake up, you will discover that you have a urinary catheter. This is because the nerve endings which normally control the bladder will have been numbed by the operation, and it can take several days for the bladder to start working again on its own. You will stay in hospital for about two weeks after the operation, and it often takes another six to eight weeks before you feel completely recovered. Before you go home, the doctors will be able to tell you the result of the microscopic examination of your uterus and lymph nodes. You will therefore be given an indication of how things are going.

Obviously, you will need to be seen regularly in the outpatient clinic, and your first appointment is usually about two months after you leave hospital. It is likely you will be asked not to have sexual intercourse until after this time.

Surgery is only possible while the cancer is still fairly localised, i.e. during the earlier stages of its development. It is the treatment of choice for young premenopausal women as it has fewer long-term side effects than radiotherapy, particularly in relation to sexual function. However, if the cancer is too advanced for surgery, or if the surgical treatment fails to clear the tumour, radiotherapy or chemotherapy need to be used.

RADIOTHERAPY

Two types of radiotherapy can be used, external and internal, the cervix being one of the few organs which is accessible enough for internal radiotherapy. Sometimes a combination of both types is used.

External radiotherapy involves short treatments with radiation (rather like a sunbed) spread over five or six weeks. Normally, the treatments are carried out from Monday to Friday, so you get a rest at weekends. In many ways, the worst part of this is the constant travelling to and from hospital, especially since nausea is a common side effect. The other side effects you may experience at the time are diarrhoea and cystitis. Bleeding sometimes occurs from the vagina both during and after the treatment but you should not let this distress you, as it is not a bad sign; it is simply the normal healing process.

Internal radiotherapy involves the insertion of a radioactive rod inside the uterus and vagina, which is left inside for between one and three days. You are given a light general anaesthetic during the actual insertion, and, unfortunately, have to be kept more or less in isolation until the element is removed. Anyone who visits you, including the nurses, have to wear protective aprons. This is because, although you cannot feel it, you are emitting some radiation from the rod, and would therefore be a hazard to other people. However, the treatment is relatively short, and there is no danger at all once it is over.

Obviously, during either type of radiotherapy, internal organs which are not in need of treatment are shielded as much as possible. However, this is never completely successful, and does result in some problems. The vagina, ovaries, bladder and bowel are most likely to be affected. The ovaries usually stop working permanently, resulting in an artificial menopause. This may be distressing but can be successfully dealt with using hormone replacement therapy. Bowel habit may be changed, resulting in either constipation or diarrhoea – usually the latter. (If mild, this is actually often viewed by women as a beneficial effect.) The bladder tends to become more sensitive, giving painful symptoms similar to cystitis. The vagina tends to shrink and stiffen, partly due to the radiation itself, and partly due to the loss of the female hormone oestrogen after the ovaries stop working. It is therefore important to resume sexual intercourse as soon as possible after treatment, to keep the vagina 'in shape'; otherwise intercourse may become very difficult later. This is one of the main reasons for avoiding radiotherapy in young women.

CHEMOTHERAPY

This involves using very powerful drugs, given either by mouth or by injection. These drugs are designed to kill cells, so they are called 'cytotoxics' ('cyto' means 'cell'). Unfortunately, they tend to kill normal cells as well as abnormal ones, so they can have unpleasant side effects, for example nausea, vomiting and hair loss. They have not been very successful yet in the treatment of cervical cancer, but may be useful in the future. At present, their use is mainly limited to very rapidly-growing cancers, prior to surgery or radiotherapy, and they may also be given after surgery if the lymph nodes are found to contain cancer cells.

RADICAL SURGERY

Removal of all the pelvic organs including the uterus, bladder and bowel (called pelvic exenteration) is occasionally used to treat advanced disease or recurrent tumours. This type of surgery is obviously a major procedure, which is only performed after very careful consideration and assessment. It is not common, and is best discussed individually with your gynaecologist, if he suggests it. It should not be confused with a Wertheim's hysterectomy, which is sometimes referred to as radical hysterectomy.

HOW SUCCESSFUL ARE THE TREATMENTS?

This depends greatly on the severity of disease. Obviously, the earlier it is treated, the better the chances of cure. If the cancer is caught at an early stage, the chances of cure can be as high as 90 per cent. However, this probability drops to about 50 per cent, or even less, if the cancer is discovered late.

Once again, it should be stressed that each individual case is different, and the information we have given can only be used as a general guide. Do not be afraid to question your gynaecologist; he or she will be the best source of information in your particular case.

7

WHAT CAUSES CERVICAL CANCER?

It has been known for over a century that cervical cancer is a sexually transmitted disease. In 1842 an Italian doctor called Rigoni-Stern noticed that nuns very rarely developed cancer of the cervix. When he looked into this further he discovered that not all nuns seemed to be 'immune' – women who had been married before entering the order seemed to be at much the same risk as the general population. He concluded that virginity was the protective factor.

SEXUAL BEHAVIOUR

His important work gathered dust for over a hundred years, until a Canadian doctor repeated the study, looking at nuns in Quebec. The confirmation of those findings opened the floodgates of research into this area in the 1950s. Suddenly everyone was interested in cervical cancer. Within a few years it had been established that the disease was particularly common in prostitutes, and that a very important risk factor was the age at which a woman first had sex; it was shown that the earlier a woman started to have sex, and the more partners she had, the greater her risk of developing cervical cancer.

Soon it was also shown that young age at first pregnancy placed a woman at risk, while women with few or no pregnancies seemed protected compared with those who had many pregnancies. Divorced, widowed or separated women were at risk. It was even shown that women who attended church regularly were less likely to develop the disease than their non-attending counterparts.

Scientists then started to look at the differences in incidence in various countries. They found that these were quite striking. Colombia had an incidence that was nearly 100 times greater than that of Israel; the United States and Europe were somewhere in between. So they turned to looking at ethnic groups. It was interesting that Jewesses tended to have the same incidence regardless of which country they lived in. The scientists then compared Jewesses, white Americans and non-white Americans who all lived in New York; non-white American women had the highest incidence, Jewesses the lowest, and white Americans were in between.

Next, it was noticed that there was a difference between the social classes, and also within each social class. (At this point we should explain that ever since the concept of 'social class' was invented, it has been assumed that a woman must belong to the same social class as her husband – not a very fair assumption nowadays.) It was found that there was a much higher incidence of cervical cancer in the lower social classes. However, regardless of social class, there was a higher incidence among women married to men whose jobs involved travel and long periods away from home, for example sailors, long-distance lorry drivers, soldiers and so on. (In Chapter 1 we drew attention to the fact that there is a space on the smear form (section 07) which is for 'Husband's occupation'. Now you know why.)

So the doctors and scientists looked at all these pieces of information and tried to find something that would link them together. The conclusion seemed inescapable; it must relate to the woman's sexual behaviour. What do prostitutes, widows, divorced women, women who marry very young, or start having sex very young have in common? They are likely to have more than one sexual partner during their lifetime. So started the 'cervical cancer is a disease of promiscuity' story. Nuns have no sexual partners, Jewesses and very religious women of any denomination tend to have only one partner – it all seemed to fit.

Then a few little contradictions started to creep in. How come cervical cancer was very common in social class 1 women in Colombia, who were usually faithful to their husbands?

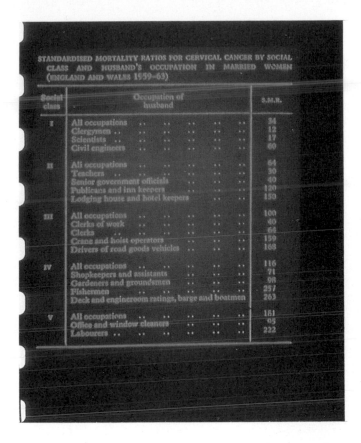

STANDARDISED MORTALITY RATIOS FOR CERVICAL CANCER BY SOCIAL
CLASS AND HUSBAND'S OCCUPATION IN MARRIED WOMEN
(ENGLAND AND WALES 1959-63)

Social class	Occupation of husband	S.M.R.
I	All occupations	34
	Clergymen	12
	Scientists	17
	Civil engineers	60
II	All occupations	54
	Teachers	30
	Senior government officials	40
	Publicans and inn keepers	120
	Lodging house and hotel keepers	150
III	All occupations	100
	Clerks of work	40
	Clerks	64
	Crane and hoist operators	159
	Drivers of road goods vehicles	168
IV	All occupations	116
	Shopkeepers and assistants	71
	Gardeners and groundsmen	98
	Fishermen	257
	Deck and engineroom ratings, barge and boatmen	263
V	All occupations	151
	Office and window cleaners	95
	Labourers	222

Risk of cervical cancer defined by husband's occupation.

07 HUSBAND'S OCCUPATION (patient's if
unmarried) also state if Manager, Foreman or other

If the patient is married, the husband's occupation is requested.

71

And who was more likely to have large numbers of sexual partners, the sailor or his wife? In the late 1960s the attention therefore turned to the men.

A very important study looked at men whose first wives had died of cervical cancer; it was found that their subsequent wives were much more likely to develop the disease. The wives of men with penile cancer were also found to have a higher incidence of cervical cancer. The sexual behaviour of men in Colombia was then studied, and it was found that the well-to-do Colombian man was accustomed to visiting prostitutes on a regular basis, while his wife remained faithful. All these studies led to the concept of the 'high-risk male', something we will discuss in greater detail in the next chapter.

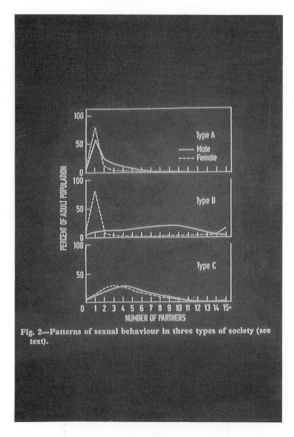

Fig. 2—Patterns of sexual behaviour in three types of society (see text).

Type A, B and C societies.

So it was not just the sexual behaviour on the part of women which was to blame – the behaviour of the men had to be taken into account as well. On the basis of the new findings, three models of behaviour could be drawn up to explain the differences in incidence between different countries, ethnic groups and religious denominations.

In a type A society both the woman and the man have only one sexual partner, i.e. each other. This is the type of behaviour found amongst religious Jews and certain other religious denominations. The incidence of cervical cancer is very low.

In type B society the woman has only one partner, but the man has many. This was the case in Colombia, and also in Victorian England. The incidence of cervical cancer is very high.

In a type C society both the man and the woman have more than one partner, but not a large number of partners. This is the general pattern of behaviour in Europe and the United States today. The incidence of cervical cancer falls above that of type A, but well below that of type B, societies.

OTHER SUSPECTED FACTORS

Having established that cervical cancer is a sexually transmitted disease, the obvious next question is 'What is it that passes between a man and a woman to cause the disease?' And it did not take long for people to start looking at sperm. It has been shown that sperm become attached to the very cells on the cervix which can eventually become abnormal. Certain types of protein, which are part of the sperm head, may be able to interfere in some way with the functions of the cell. However, the exact mechanism is still unknown and the effect is only a weak one, although it is possible that these so-called basic proteins may 'help' some other agent to cause abnormalities in cells. Also, one study has already shown that the wart virus (to be discussed in the next chapter) can be passed on through semen.

The next suggestion was that it might be something to do with personal hygiene. This was based mainly on the fact that there was a low incidence among Jews, who are circumcised. Perhaps smegma, the substance which collects under the foreskin, had something to do with it? This idea of personal hygiene seemed to tie in well with the social class variation. A man coming home after a long day's work at the coal face might well be more 'dirty' than an office clerk. Unfortunately for this theory, the facts just did not add up. For example, there is a tribe in Malaysia which still lives in a very primitive fashion. The men are uncircumcised, the girls marry at about fourteen years old, and they have never heard of the idea of hygiene. In addition, the women start having children immediately after their marriage and tend to have a large number. Despite all this, their incidence of cervical cancer is very low. Of more significance is the fact that they do not have premarital sex, and remain faithful to each other after marriage. As we have already seen, this is also the more likely explanation for the low incidence of cervical cancer amongst Jews.

In recent years smoking has become a focus of attention. Heavy smokers (over 20 cigarettes a day) seem to be up to seven times at risk compared to non-smokers. The reasons for this are still unclear. However, nicotine has been found in very high concentrations in the cervical cells of smokers, and it is thought that nicotine damages the cells' immune responses and so makes them more susceptible to other forms of infection, such as the wart virus for example (see Chapter 8).

THE PILL

The likelihood of contracting cervical cancer also seems to be influenced by the type of contraception a woman uses. Barrier methods of contraception, such as the sheath and, to a lesser extent, the diaphragm, seem to have a protective effect. This is not surprising, since they offer protection against a number of sexually transmitted diseases. Neither the IUD (coil), nor the progestogen only pill (POP, or mini-pill) have been shown to have any effect on the incidence of cervical cancer.

The combined oral contraceptive pill, though, has been the subject of much controversy in relation to cervical cancer. Some studies have shown no effect, but others have shown a small increase in risk if a woman is taking this type of pill. It is very difficult to reach any definite conclusions either way, mainly because of the number of other factors which could influence the results of the studies. For example, the vast majority of studies do not take into account the number of sexual partners of the male. As we have seen earlier in this chapter (and will show again in Chapter 8), this aspect is actually very important. And there are other factors which could bias the results; for example, are women on the pill more likely to be in steady relationships and therefore having sex more often? Or are they more likely to have a larger number of sexual partners? Are they more likely to smoke? Although the trend in the last few years has been away from smoking if you are on the pill, remember these studies look at women who were taking the pill ten or fifteen years ago, when the risks were not appreciated, and smoking was fashionable. In addition, the women studied were taking high-dose pills, which are rarely used today.

A large World Health Organisation study, published in 1985, showed a relative risk of only 1.19 for women taking high-dose pills. This relative risk increased to 1.53 after five years of pill use. They did not ask about smoking habits, or the number of sexual partners of the male. Whatever risk there is, then, must be small. And it is as well to remember in this context that pregnancy is one of the high-risk factors for cervical cancer; the pill gives 99.5 per cent protection against pregnancy (considerably better than almost all the other reversible methods of contraception), so it is performing a useful function in this respect. So, if the alternative to being on the pill is being pregnant, you are better off on the pill.

For this reason, a woman need not stop the pill, even if she has a positive smear, and she can carry on taking the pill after her cervix has been treated. Obviously, a 'belt and braces' approach would be to take the pill for contraception and to use a barrier method as well, to give added protection to the cervix.

PREGNANCY AND ADOLESCENCE

Let's now take another look at the cervix itself. We've already mentioned that both sex and pregnancy in adolescence seem to be risk factors. In addition, pregnancy at any age seems to be a risk factor. Do pregnancy and adolescence have anything in common? The answer is yes. During both pregnancy and adolescence a great deal of activity goes on in the transformation zone; as you will remember from Chapter 2 it is in this area that soft columnar cells change to become hard squamous cells – squamous metaplasia. This is a perfectly normal process, but it is at this time that cells are most vulnerable to any outside influences which might cause them to develop in an abnormal way. In both pregnancy and adolescence, this squamous metaplasia goes on at a much faster rate and involves a larger number of cells. This means that there are more cells around which are vulnerable to attack, and also that the whole process of abnormal change can take place more quickly. It has been known for some time that dysplasia (development of abnormal changes in cells) can progress more quickly in pregnancy, and therefore needs very careful monitoring.

GENETIC FACTORS

In recent years some evidence has emerged which suggests that certain women may be genetically more at risk of getting cervical cancer. First, a study showed that the cervical mucus of a woman with cervical cancer was deficient in a particular type of enzyme called antitrypsin. Trypsin is an 'attacking enzyme', so this would suggest that these women's cells had weaker defence systems; in this way they might be more vulnerable to attack by any cancer-inducing substance or agent. The presence and amount of an enzyme in the body is determined by a gene (inheritable material), which codes specifically for it, so the conclusion drawn from this evidence is that these women have a different genetic make-up from those who do not get cervical cancer. Another study has shown that women who have more than the usual numbers of a particular type of gene are much more likely to develop invasive cancer than those who have the normal amount. This area of study is really only just beginning; it will be a long time before it can be of any practical use.

VIRUSES

In the 1960s, however, scientists everywhere were searching for a sexually transmitted 'agent' that could be the cause of cervical cancer. The idea of viruses being a cause of cancer was one that had long been popular, so it was not surprising that attention soon turned to them. The next chapter deals with this, perhaps most significant, part of the story.

8

VIRUSES AND CERVICAL CANCER

WHAT IS A VIRUS?

Louis Pasteur and his pupil, Emile Roux, were the first scientists to show that something even smaller than bacteria could cause disease in both animals and man. Their work on the rabies virus in the 1880s paved the way for years of intensive research into viruses. The microscopes in use at that time were not powerful enough to show up any kind of virus, so these micro-organisms were, in effect, completely invisible. Scientists could only guess at what they might be like.

There was only one way to study the effects of a virus; a solution made from diseased tissue was passed through a very fine filter, with holes so small that no ordinary cells or bacteria could get through. This filtered solution was then injected into an animal; the animal still developed the disease, showing that a disease-causing agent remained in the solution after it was filtered.

That was all well and good, but they still did not know what it was about the solutions that caused disease. The major breakthrough did not come until 1935, when an American scientist, Wendell Stanley, managed to form crystals from a solution. When he redissolved the crystals in water, they still caused disease. This made it look as though viruses were not alive at all but just complicated proteins.

The next big step forward was the discovery that viruses contained either RNA (ribonucleic acid) or DNA (deoxyribonucleic acid). As their names suggest, these substances are found in the nucleus of a cell. They are the inheritable material that make up the genes which decide what type of cell it will be, and what it will do.

A virus uses its own DNA or RNA to take over control of the cell, usurping the function of the cell's DNA and RNA, and using the cell to reproduce itself. (However, some viruses may simply enter the cell and lie dormant for long periods of time; this is true of the human papilloma virus, which we shall be discussing in detail later.) Viruses therefore cannot exist without a host cell to provide for their needs; in this they are different from bacteria, which are self-sufficient entities in their own right.

This invasion by viruses does not go unopposed, however. A type of white blood cell manufactures proteins which are designed *specifically* to fight that particular virus. They travel in the bloodstream and are called antibodies. This is an important concept, because it is these antibodies which form the basis of immunity. Once created, a number of them will always be present. If the same micro-organism, e.g. virus, or foreign body tries to invade again, these proteins can be reproduced very quickly and provide a very strong defence. By the same token, doctors can tell if a person has had a certain type of infection in the past by checking their blood for the specific antibody against that infection. (You may, for example, have been checked for antibodies against German measles, to decide whether you needed the vaccine.) We will be mentioning this again later.

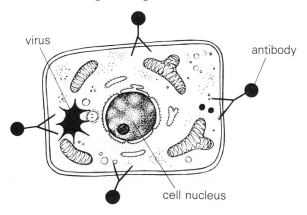

The immune response involves antibodies which latch on to a cell after a virus has invaded it.

VIRUSES AND CANCER

At first, scientists only looked to see if viruses caused infectious diseases, like bacteria, but in 1911 another French scientist, Rous, demonstrated that a filtered solution could produce cancer in birds. This was the beginning of what proved to be a rapidly expanding area of research. Indeed, people began to think that viruses were the cause of *all* cancers.

Numerous examples of viral cancers started to be found in animals. A virus was found to cause leukemia in cats, another to cause skin cancer in rabbits, yet another to cause breast cancer in mice. The list is very long and continues to grow. And human cancers increasingly became associated with viruses. For example, the virus which causes a type of glandular fever may occasionally also cause cancer of the nasal passages and a type of lymphoma (cancer of the lymph nodes). Another example is provided by one of the viruses which causes hepatitis, and which can also cause cancer of the liver.

It seemed obvious, therefore, to search for a viral cause of cervical cancer. In fact, viruses of several kinds are not too difficult to find in cervical cancer or pre-cancer tissue; the problem is to show that they are not just 'innocent bystanders'. This is an important distinction; by way of analogy, just because someone happens to be found at the scene of a crime does not automatically mean he is guilty of murder.

There have been three main contenders for the role of 'the cervical cancer virus'. These are, in order of probable importance, human papilloma virus, herpes simplex virus and cytomegalovirus. We will consider each of them in turn.

CYTOMEGALOVIRUS

This is a very common virus. It may cause a flu-like illness, or even, occasionally, a type of glandular fever, but most people are quite unaware that they have had the infection. If caught in pregnancy it can be dangerous because it can affect the baby (rather like German measles).

Cytomegalovirus (CMV) can also be sexually transmitted, and has been found in tissue from the cervix, as well as in semen. This fact led to suspicion that it might be causing cervical cancer. Indeed, it was found to be present more often in cervical cancer than in normal tissue. However, it is so common that it is difficult to explain why more women have not developed cancer. It is also quite possible that, once cells have become weakened by the real cancer agent, CMV makes the most of an easy opportunity to invade. It seems unlikely though that CMV will prove to be important in the causation of cervical cancer.

HERPES SIMPLEX VIRUS

If this book had been written ten years ago, we would have been very excited about the herpes simplex virus (HSV) – such is the passing nature of fame. However, it is interesting to look at the herpes story; indeed, there may be some life in the theory yet.

There are two kinds of herpes virus, HSV 1, which usually causes cold sores, and HSV 2, which usually causes genital herpes (although occasionally they can swap over). It is HSV 2 we are mainly interested in.

The herpes virus was already known to be capable of causing kidney tumours in frogs. In addition, it is a close relative of the glandular fever virus, mentioned above, which is associated with two types of cancer in humans. Around 1966 it was noticed that women who suffered from genital herpes seem to have more than their fair share of abnormal smears. Scientists therefore started looking for antibodies to HSV 2 in women with cervical cancer. (We mentioned antibodies on page 80. If a person has antibodies to a virus in their blood, it means that at some point they have been infected with that virus. It is like a fingerprint left behind long after the culprit has gone.) The scientists found that a high proportion of women with cervical cancer had these antibodies, while a group of women who were similar, but did not have cancer, were found to be much less likely to have such antibodies. This looked very promising.

Unfortunately, as more and more studies were done, so large discrepancies started to appear. The proportion of women with cervical cancer who had antibodies to HSV 2 could vary from as high as 90 per cent to as low as 30 per cent.

Herpes is a highly infectious disease, and it was quite possible that these figures simply reflected the level of infection in a given area. The studies were, after all, being done during the 'swinging sixties' and early 1970s, when liberated attitudes resulted in an increase in all forms of sexually transmitted disease.

In the 1970s researchers started to look at the activity of viruses after they had actually got inside the cells. As we mentioned earlier, viruses are made up of genetic material, in the form of DNA or RNA; some viruses incorporate their own DNA into that of the cell and in this way the cell's 'blueprint' is changed and the virus takes control. However when scientists looked at cells which had been attacked by the herpes virus, they found that very little, if any, of this incorporation had taken place. The virus seemed to have damaged the cells in various ways, but did not appear to have taken control. It seemed that the herpes virus was behaving in a 'hit and run' fashion. This makes it much less likely that the herpes virus could be an important cause of cervical cancer on its own. However, by damaging the cells, it makes them more vulnerable to any further attack, so it may act as a 'primer' for a more important agent.

As scientists began to be disillusioned with the herpes theory, they started to notice that the wart, or human papilloma virus (HPV) was often found in cervical cancer tissue. Could this be the virus they had been looking for?

THE HUMAN PAPILLOMA VIRUS (HPV)

It had been known since 1907 that warts could be transmitted by a cell-free solution, i.e. by some sort of submicroscopic infecting agent. Then, in 1933, it was shown that the wart virus caused skin cancer in cotton-tail rabbits. However an interesting feature which emerged was that the wart virus did not always cause cancer; it seemed to need 'help' from some other source. For example, a wart virus causes gut cancer in cows, but only if they also eat bracken. Sheep infected with the wart virus can get skin cancer, but only in parts of the body which are directly exposed to sunlight.

In the late 1970s workers started to look at cells which had been infected with the wart virus, and they found that there was not just one type of wart virus, but many different types, identified by the type of DNA they contained. Although they were all related, they seemed to behave quite differently; for example, the type which causes plantar warts (the common verruca) shows little interest in infecting cervical cells. In addition, while some types of wart virus could be found in cervical cells, not all of them were actually incorporated into the cells' DNA, so again it appeared that some were just 'innocent bystanders'.

As research technology became more sophisticated, it was possible to work out the exact types of wart virus which were present in different places. Currently, there are over forty different types of wart virus, and the number identified is growing all the time. Type 1 is the verruca virus. The genital warts which you can see on the vulva or the penis are usually caused by types 6 or 11, and these types are also often seen in cervical cells, although they do not seem to be incorporated into the cells' DNA. However, when types 16 or 18 are found in cervical cells, they *are* usually incorporated into the DNA, and it is these two types which are most often found in cervical cancer.

So it looks as though there are low-risk wart viruses (e.g. types 6 and 11) and high-risk viruses (types 16 and 18). The trouble is that both low-risk and high-risk types can cause cell changes. It is not possible to tell which is which from a cervical smear, or even a biopsy, unless special techniques are used to look at the DNA in the cells. At present the process is expensive and time-consuming, so it is only done in the few hospitals which are interested in research.

When a cell is invaded by a wart virus, characteristic changes can be seen under the microscope. These changes are not actually part of the pre-cancer spectrum, and the cells which show signs of wart virus invasion are called koilocytes. This is a term you may see cropping up on smear reports from time to time. Another way it may be written is 'HPV infection seen'. Wart virus changes can in fact be seen as a characteristic appearance during colposcopy. Biopsies taken during colposcopy will also show the wart virus, and can be used to find out which type of wart virus is present. The herpes virus can cause changes in cells, too (as mentioned above), but these again look different. If the changes are obviously due to herpes, this will be indicated in section 22.

Fold

Some cells show koilocytosis.

23 EVIDENCE OF NEOPLASIA CYTOLOGICAL PATTERN SUGGESTS:		24 INFLAMMATION		25 FURTHER INVESTIGATION SUGGESTED	
Inadequate specimen	1	Severe Inflammatory Change	1	Repeat smear in months	1
Negative	2	Trichomonas	2	or after treatment	2
Mild dysplasia	3	Candida	4	Colposcopy 16	
Severe dysplasia/ carcinoma-in-situ	4	Viral	(8)	Cervical biopsy	4
				Uterine curettage 8	
Carcinoma-in-situ/? invasive	5	Signature		date	
? Glandular neoplasia	6	*Fold*			

Smear form result showing viral damage.

In addition to changes that can be seen in cells, antibodies are formed to the specific type of wart virus or viruses which have caused the infection, and these antibodies can be detected in blood samples. About 90 per cent of women with cervical cancer have antibodies to HPV, while antibodies to HPV have also been found in about 95 per cent of people who have genital warts. In addition about 60 per cent of women with CIN have antibodies to HPV. However, when a group of women with neither warts, nor cervical cancer, nor CIN were studied, virtually none had antibodies to HPV.

All this evidence implicates the wart virus as a major cause of cervical cancer. Another important study looked at a group of women who had CIN 1, the first stage of cellular abnormality or pre-cancer. The women were carefully assessed over a period of about two years, during which time about a quarter progressed to CIN 3. We will be mentioning this study again later, but for the present let us just look at the presence of the wart virus in these women. More than half of them had HPV 6 (a low-risk virus), while about a third had HPV 16 (a high-risk virus). Some, of course, had both, which makes the actual equations more complicated. The interesting thing is that, although HPV 16 was the less common type overall, it was present in 85 per cent of the women whose disease progressed. This is strong evidence suggesting not only that the wart virus is a cause of cervical cancer, but also that only certain types of the virus (in this study, HPV 16) are involved.

So where does this wart virus come from? To answer that question, several studies have been done looking at men. One looked at a group of men whose partners had CIN. Over two-thirds of them were found to have wart virus infection of the penis. Not all of them had visible warts, however; nearly half had infections which only showed up when acetic acid was used, just as in colposcopy. (Areas which have wart virus infection show up with acetic acid and have a characteristic appearance.)

Now, of course, it could be argued that the men got their infection from their female partners. However, studies have gone on to show that women who previously had normal smears and showed no signs of wart virus infection are more likely to develop both warts and CIN if they have a long-term faithful relationship with a man who has warts.

This fits in well with the concept of the high-risk male, which we first mentioned in Chapter 7. Men may, in fact, be unaware they have a high-risk virus infection. The problem is that, as we mentioned earlier, the HPV types which cause visible warts (types 6 and 11) are not actually the important ones as far as cervical cancer is concerned. It is the invisible ones, types 16 and 18, which are to blame. Men who have visible warts may have other areas of wart virus infection with types 16 and 18, of which they, their partners and their doctors are quite unaware. These areas will only show up if they are painted with acetic acid. Similarly, men who have no visible warts at all may still have wart virus infection. Unfortunately, treatment is only available for visible warts, as it is usually impractical (and painful) to try and treat large areas of essentially normal skin.

Why isn't there an epidemic of penile cancer if so many men are infected? The answer lies in the difference between the cells on the cervix and the penis. In Chapter 2 we mentioned that the vulnerable area on the cervix is the transformation zone, where soft columnar cells change into hard, squamous cells. Cells which are in the process of change can be easily attacked by the wart virus. However, no such change occurs in the cells of the penis. The cells there are all tough squamous cells, and are very resistant to attack. Penile cancer is very rare indeed.

Another question which springs to mind is 'Why don't all women with warts develop cervical cancer?' Part of the answer is likely to be the fact that only certain types of HPV are dangerous. However, to confuse matters even more, not even all the women who have the high-risk HPV types 16 and 18 develop cancer. In addition, in some people both warts and CIN disappear without any treatment. What is it that makes them special?

You may remember that, earlier in this chapter, we mentioned that whenever warts cause cancer, they seem to need help from some other source. An interesting observation has been that people whose immune system is not functioning well seem to be particularly prone to warts. This was noticed in people who are on strong treatments for other cancers, and also in people who have kidney transplants; the latter have to have their immune system suppressed so that they do not reject their new kidney. Pregnancy is also a time when warts can become rampant and are very difficult to get rid of – and it has long been known that CIN progresses much faster in pregnancy. More recently, it has been noticed that people with AIDS are much more prone to warts – their basic problem is also a suppression of their immune system.

So, anything which weakens the body's immune system makes it easier for the wart virus to invade. For example, smoking has been shown to affect the cells which form an important part of the immune defences, and this adverse effect seems to be particularly strong in the cells of the cervix. Similarly, men who smoke have been shown to be more likely to have wart virus infection of the penis, while women who smoke have up to ten times the normal risk of developing cervical cancer. The obvious inference from all this is that smoking weakens the cells' defences and thus allows the wart virus to take hold. Similarly, the herpes virus, by damaging the cells during its attack, may make it easier for a later invasion by the wart virus.

Smoking and herpes are only two possible sources of help for the wart virus; there may be many others. Sperm proteins, mentioned in Chapter 7, may also act in this way. There is a lot of research still going on in this area.

PROTECTION AND TREATMENT

Is there any way you can protect yourself from warts? Well, it would certainly seem sensible to avoid smoking yourself, and possibly even avoid men who smoke. Remember that you can't necessarily tell if they are infected just by looking. Condoms do offer protection against most sexually transmitted diseases, and the diaphragm also offers some protection.

Any woman who has had warts or herpes herself, or is the partner of a man who has either of these infections, should have yearly smears. That way, if any abnormal cell changes do occur, they will be discovered early and treated before they become serious.

Both men and women who develop genital warts are often very upset at the inference that they must have been unfaithful to have got a sexually transmitted disease – especially since they are quite often in a long-term monogamous relationship. The answer to this fraught question lies in the incubation period of warts. The virus can lie dormant in the cells for years before any visible warts actually appear; no-one knows their maximum incubation period. This means that wart virus caught during a relationship many years in the past may suddenly surface.

If viruses are a risk factor for cervical cancer, is there any way of getting rid of them before pre-cancerous changes occur? Similarly, will the virus still be there after treatment for pre-cancer? These questions are uppermost in the minds of doctors and scientists in this field.

Viruses in fact are very difficult to kill, since they are only susceptible when they are reproducing; often the only way to eliminate them is to kill the cells which are supporting them. If they have invaded a large number of cells, treatment aimed at eliminating the virus might actually kill the person as well.

So far, no treatment has been found which eradicates viruses completely and permanently. For example, a drug called acyclovir is useful in the treatment of a herpes attack. It stops the replication of the herpes virus in infected cells, but leaves normal uninfected cells untouched. It therefore has very few side effects. Unfortunately, because it only affects cells in which the virus is replicating, it has no effect on cells where the virus is lying dormant, so it is only a matter of time before these surface and cause another attack.

Local treatments for warts all suffer the disadvantage that, obviously, they will only work where they are applied. As we have seen, the wart virus may be present in cells without causing visible warts; indeed, the more dangerous types are precisely the ones which are 'invisible'. This does not mean, however, that the visible warts should be ignored. They can grow to quite enormous sizes and look very unpleasant. The visible warts also act as a warning sign of possible risk to the cervix; a third of women who have visible genital warts also have CIN. The high-risk wart viruses seem to travel alongside the low-risk ones, so it is common to be infected with both types at the same time.

There are several local treatments for warts. The ones most commonly used are the paints, based on a compound called podophyllum, available as Podophyllin paint. An acid, trichloracetic acid, is also used, but only very carefully, as it can cause burns. Both laser treatment and cryotherapy (discussed fully in Chapter 5) can be used to treat warts, but, again, they are unlikely to eradicate the virus completely. It is difficult to say which treatment is best; one of the major problems in any study is that warts often go away on their own, only to return later, so it can be difficult to tell whether it was, in fact, the treatment which made them go away.

A new local treatment is beginning to emerge which may prove useful. It is based on a very strong drug called 5 fluorouracil. It is given by injection in cancer chemotherapy, but has also been made into a cream, which is how it could be useful for treatment of wart-infected cells. It seems to kill infected cells without harming normal ones. This means it can, for example, be applied all over the vulva and inserted into the vagina. Invisible wart virus infection could be eradicated in this way, and it might even be possible to use it on penile skin as well, to try and get rid of the 'reservoir' of infection in men. It does, however, cause skin irritation, and it cannot be used in pregnancy as it would harm the foetus. It is gradually coming into use, and is being studied all the time.

A second cancer chemotherapy drug is also being tried. It is called bleomycin, and is injected, in very small doses, into warts. It seems to be quite successful in treating warts which have resisted all other forms of treatment, and, so far, appears to have few side effects.

We have mentioned that a person's immune system is

important in keeping the wart virus at bay. Various treatments have therefore been looked at which might boost this immune response. So far, the one most studied has been interferon. Interferon is a substance which the body produces as part of its defence against viruses. In theory, injecting more of it should improve the defence. Unfortunately, the side effects have been so bad that its use is very limited at present. It needs to be given by injection for several months, during which time the person feels extremely ill, as if they have a bad dose of flu. Injecting individual warts with interferon has also been tried, with some success and a slight improvement in side effects. Research is continuing in this area, but it is unlikely to be a major help in the near future.

Another drug, which also aims to stimulate the body's immune response, is being tried in both herpes and wart virus research. It is called inosine pranobex (or Immunovir). So far, it has not been very successful in herpes, but the initial trials seem to show some benefit against warts. It will be years yet before we really know either way.

As you can see, there is a long way to go before we can be really sure of the cause or causes of cervical cancer. However, there *is* a strong association with the wart virus, and this theory is the most promising and exciting to date. It does seem fairly certain that there is no one cause, but several, acting together. Treatment is unlikely to offer certain cure, nor will future protection be guaranteed until we know the causes and can treat both the male and female partners. (However, you should remember that treatment for cervical pre-cancer has a 90 to 95 per cent cure rate, despite the fact that we cannot be sure all the virus has been eradicated.)

The only thing that can be done in the interim is to screen women as thoroughly as possible. If we cannot offer certain protection against pre-cancer, at least we should be able to prevent the progression to cancer. The next chapter discusses how this can be done, and why it is not always happening at present.

9

HOW OFTEN TO HAVE A SMEAR?

Cervical cancer is unique in that it has well-defined pre-cancerous stages that can easily be diagnosed and treated. In theory, therefore, it should be possible to eradicate the disease almost completely. Why is it, then, that worldwide nearly half a million new cases of cervical cancer are diagnosed every year?

WHO IS AT RISK?

First of all, let us look at just who is dying of cervical cancer. There are in fact two major groups. The biggest group is of women over the age of 45 who have never had a cervical smear. However, the other important and ever-increasing group is of young women under the age of 35.

About 80 per cent of women who develop cervical cancer are over the age of 40, and nearly all of them have never had a smear. It is one of the problems of any attempt at screening that the people who are most at risk are the least likely to come for tests. Older women often have the mistaken impression that by attending for a smear they will be viewed as having been promiscuous. They also belong to a generation which is not used to health screening and therefore do not look on it as part of their routine health care. Lack of understanding generates fear – women who do not understand what a smear test is are sometimes afraid that if it is abnormal they must already have cancer, and it is only a small psychological step from this point of view to a feeling that they would rather not know. A great deal of health education is needed before such misconceptions can be corrected.

The other group which is causing concern is the small but rapidly increasing number of young women who are developing cervical cancer. Since the mid-1960s the percentage has increased from 2 per cent to 20 per cent. It is also worrying that the disease seems to progress faster in young women, so they have less chance of being caught in time.

It is often said that far too many smears are taken from young women, who are supposedly at low risk. However, this ten-fold increase in cervical cancer in women under 35 has occurred *despite* the fact that they are having so many smears. What would have happened if they had not had them?

There is evidence that we are about to experience a virtual epidemic of cervical cancer. Between 1973 and 1979 there was a 117 per cent increase in the number of pre-cancers, but only an 11 per cent increase in the number of smears taken. This increase in pre-cancers has been greatest in young women; in older women the numbers are actually falling slightly. So why is there such a different pattern?

To understand what the graph opposite is telling us, we must look at what is called the 'cohort effect'. As you can see, it looks from the graph as if there has been a large drop in the incidence of cancer in the 45–54-year-old age group, and it is often assumed that this is due to screening. However, this is only part of the story.

Women who were about 60 in the mid-1970s were born around the time of the First World War, and were therefore in their 20s during the Second World War. This was a time when wives were separated from their husbands, when young lovers did not know if they would see each other again, when soldiers arrived in communities and then moved on. This, coupled with the feeling that 'we might all be dead tomorrow', resulted in a less strict code of sexual behaviour. As a result of their promiscuity, these women as a group (or cohort) are at high risk of developing cervical cancer.

However, the group of women who are now 40 to 50 years old were born just before or during the Second World War, and reached their 'dating' years in the mid-1950s. This was a time of strict parental control and moral attitudes, so neither they nor their partners were likely to become sexually active

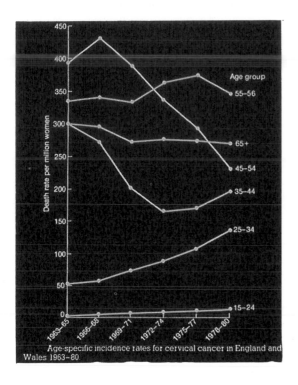

Age-specific incidence rates for cervical cancer in England and Wales 1963–80.

Age of incidence of cervical cancer.

very early, or have multiple partners. As a result, despite being at a high-risk age, these women are in fact a relatively low-risk group. This is the explanation for the apparent decrease in incidence shown on the graph.

Young women now, brought up in the aftermath of the 'swinging sixties', are a high-risk group. Sexual liberation has brought with it an increase in sexually transmitted diseases of all kinds, including herpes and genital warts; even if the pendulum swings right back because of AIDS, because of their exposure to high-risk factors they will continue to carry this risk throughout their lives.

As we mentioned earlier, the incidence of cervical cancer in young women has already increased ten-fold. This increase is likely to continue. It is therefore important that young women should have regular cervical smears. In addition, educating young women while they are still likely to be receptive to advice is the best way to ensure that they continue to have smears as they get older. Persuading older women to come for screening tests they have not experienced before is more of a problem – you can't teach an old dog new tricks.

WHY HAVE REGULAR SMEAR TESTS?

There is no doubt that the use of cervical smears, if properly organised, will lead to a reduction in cervical cancer. Countries such as Iceland, and the province of British Columbia in Canada, have shown dramatic falls in incidence since they introduced organised screening programmes. There has been much debate about who should be screened and how often they should be screened. In practice, the arguments are only about money, because the answers to these questions have been known since the mid-1970s.

Months since last negative smear	Relative protection
0–11	15.3
12–23	11.9
24–35	8.0
36–47	5.3
48–59	2.8
Never screened	1.0

Effectiveness of regular smear testing.

The figures in this table are taken from a large international study published in 1986 – the latest in a long line of studies which have shown similar results. All the numbers are compared with the woman who has never been screened; she is the standard, with no added protection, so is designated as 1.0. The woman who has yearly smears is about 12 times better protected, but the woman who has five-yearly smears is only three times better protected. It follows that yearly screening is considerably more effective at protecting against cervical cancer than is five-yearly screening.

In Chapter 2, and indeed throughout this book, we have stressed that cervical cell changes take a long time to develop into actual cancer. Yet here we are saying that a couple of years between smears makes a difference. The two pieces of information may sound contradictory, but they are both true. The problem lies with the smear test itself. A negative smear is not always a negative smear. In fact, the false negative rate in the presence of abnormal cells has been shown to reach as high as 50 per cent. There are a number of reasons for this.

Firstly, the fault may be in the technique of taking the smear. Obviously, if the spatula is not wiped across the cervix, the result will be quite meaningless. Similarly, part of the cervix may be missed, and it may be precisely that part which has abnormal cells. In Chapter 1 we discussed the various types of spatula that have been developed to make smears more accurate. In particular, the cytobrush is very useful for picking up cells from the endocervical canal, which are often missed by a spatula. And the woman who is having the smear test done has a part to play in making sure the smear is accurate. If you are very tense, it can be extremely difficult – sometimes impossible – to take an accurate smear. The doctor or nurse may make the best of a bad job, but it is you who suffer in the end through not having an accurate smear.

Secondly, mistakes can happen in the cytology laboratory. Looking down a microscope at slides all day, every day, is incredibly boring. Mistakes are bound to happen occasionally, through poor concentration; for example it has been shown that slides which are looked at on Monday morning or Friday afternoon are more likely to be misinterpreted.

And there is a more worrying aspect to misinterpretation of slides. It has been shown that if two different cytologists look at the same slide, they are quite likely to grade it differently. Indeed, the same cytologist can give a different opinion on the same slide on different days. Such is the confusion in this field that a scientific paper has made the comment that cytology is 'a matter of opinion rather than fact'.

What this all boils down to is that single smear results, taken in isolation, are not always reliable. However, it is very unlikely that a succession of negative smears taken from the same woman will all be false negatives, which is why it is important not to leave lengthy intervals between smears. For example, if a woman is having yearly smears, an occasional false negative result is unlikely to matter; she will have an accurate smear within a year or two, which should be well in time to show up an abnormality before it becomes a cancer. However if the same woman is only having a smear once every five years, the situation is quite different. If she has a false negative smear, there is then a ten-year gap between her last real negative smear and the date her next smear is due. This is too long, and she may then find that she does have cancer, despite having had a 'negative' smear within the last five years.

If you look again at the table on page 94, you will notice that, although there is not a great deal of difference in protection between yearly and two-yearly screening, by the time three-yearly screening is reached the level of protection is halved. So three-yearly screening is really the maximum interval which should be left between smears. Obviously, yearly smears are the ideal. However, a good compromise is as follows; yearly smears until there are two completely negative ones in a row, and then two-yearly smears thereafter. This minimises the effect of the false negative smear, without the need for yearly smears all the time. However it should be stressed that this does *not* apply to women with risk factors such as genital warts or herpes, or any woman who has ever had an abnormal smear; these women should *always* have yearly smears.

And when should a woman begin having smears? Various suggestions have been made; at the age of 35, at the age of 20, in the first pregnancy, on starting the pill, etc. These are all misguided. A woman needs to have a smear within a year or two of her first experience of sexual intercourse. The age is irrelevant; she may be 16, 20, 35, 45 . . . And once she has started to have smears, she should have them at regular intervals as discussed above.

Where can a woman go to have her smear? General practitioners are the traditional source of screening. However, family planning clinics, well woman clinics and sexually transmitted disease clinics (special clinics) provide a good screening service and do not require referral from another doctor. Some women are embarrassed to have gynaecological examinations by their GP, especially if he is male and/or has known them since childhood.

IS THE SMEAR RESULT ACCURATE?

Having a smear taken is one thing, getting hold of the result is another. Women often forget when and where they last had a smear. Sometimes they have had a smear during a gynaecological check-up, but are unaware that it was done. This may lead to unnecessary duplication of smears, but may also result in a situation where smears are assumed to have been taken when in fact they were not. Some clinics and GPs give to each woman a personalised 'cervical smear record card' so she knows the date and result of her last smear. In the last few

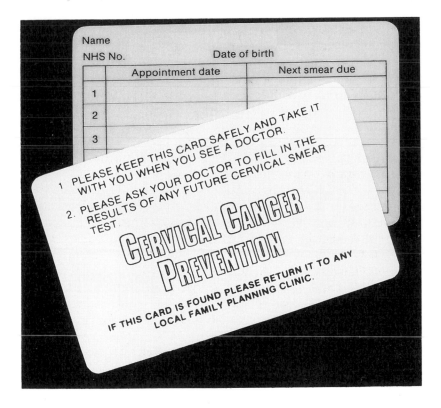

Cervical smear record cards.

years there has been considerable publicity regarding women who, for one reason or another, did not receive their smear results, as a result of which they did not have follow-up checks and subsequently died of cancer. It is up to you to make sure you know when you last had a smear and to find out what the result was. After all, it is your life that may be at risk. It is a mistake to rely on other people to take this important responsibility. They may be dealing with thousands of results; you are only interested in one, your own. Who is the more likely to lose it?

Having read this book, you should be in a position to understand what your smear result means. If you have a smear showing any degree of dyskaryosis (i.e. cell changes) you should be referred for colposcopy. In the past, and unfortunately sometimes at present, abnormal smears were simply repeated at varying intervals. Nothing was done until the smear showed severe dyskaryosis (dysplasia). In theory this should have been all right, because there should still have been time to deal with the problem. Unfortunately, this is where another limitation of the smear test comes to light.

It has been shown that smears are simply not an accurate indicator of the degree of abnormality present. So, for example, a smear report of mild dysplasia may turn out to be CIN 3 on biopsy. This means that the practice of waiting for the results to get worse is wrong; by the time they have got worse it may be too late. The reasons for inaccurate smear reports are much the same as those for false negative reports: the most important area of the cervix may not have been sampled; it may have been a Friday afternoon; or the cytologist may have had an 'off day'.

It has often been said that mild degrees of dysplasia are likely to improve on their own. This is the basis of the philosophy of simply repeating mildly abnormal smears in the hope that they will become normal in time; some women have had abnormal smears at six-monthly intervals for two or three years. However there is now plenty of evidence to say that such an approach cannot be justified. For a start, we have just pointed out that a smear is not a reliable indication of the degree of abnormality present. In addition, remember how high the false negative rate can be. If an abnormal smear is followed by a negative smear, how sure can you be that it is a true result?

An important study looked at 100 women who had CIN 1 proven by colposcopy. This would be equivalent to mild dysplasia on their smear. They were monitored for just under two years, to see what would happen. During that time, 26 of the women developed CIN 3. In 67 women there was no significant change in the degree of abnormality, and only seven women had no evidence of abnormality at the end of the study. This study was particularly important because no biopsies were taken. There have been studies which have shown higher regression rates, but they all took biopsies from the abnormal areas. As you might expect, if a large proportion of the abnormality is removed by the biopsy, the disease is bound to improve or progress more slowly. Indeed, it is thought that taking a biopsy stimulates the immune system and is therefore almost like a treatment in itself.

WHEN SHOULD YOU HAVE A COLPOSCOPY?

As you saw from the results above, only a tiny proportion of abnormal cell changes improve on their own. What is more, over a quarter had turned into severe abnormalities within two years. This means that every woman who has an abnormal smear, regardless of the actual degree of abnormality, should have a colposcopy.

Take note of this appalling, but true story. Suzanne, a 35-year-old woman, went to see her general practitioner in May 1977, complaining of a vaginal discharge. A cervical smear taken at the time showed 'atypical squamous cells'. She had a repeat smear taken in May 1978, which was negative. Four years later she again had a vaginal discharge and went to see her GP. This time the smear report read 'widespread dyskaryosis and trichomoniasis'. Trichomonas is a common sexually transmitted infection, which can show up on a smear. She was given a course of antibiotics. In January 1985 she was bleeding between her periods and also after intercourse. She was referred to a gynaecologist, who noticed she had a cervical erosion (see Chapter 3 for an explanation of this term). This can be a cause of bleeding after intercourse, so he decided to treat the erosion by cryotherapy (freezing). She bled so heavily after this procedure that she had to have a blood transfusion. By June of the same year all her symptoms had returned; she was again bleeding between periods and after intercourse. A smear was taken, which showed 'severe dyskaryosis and unusual squamous cells'. At this point she was referred, not for a colposcopy, but for a cone biopsy. Suzanne was completely unaware that she had had a succession of abnormal smears during the last eight years. She was shocked and surprised by this sudden news. She refused to have the cone biopsy and instead insisted on a referral for colposcopy. Colposcopy and biopsy revealed that she had invasive cancer of the cervix, which had already progressed to quite a late stage. In September 1985 she had a hysterectomy. At operation it was found that her abdominal lymph nodes were already invaded by the cancer. Suzanne died in July 1986.

If Suzanne had had a colposcopy after her first, or even her second, abnormal smear she would be alive today. Her case is not unique; it illustrates how careless the management of abnormal smears can be. It also demonstrates the importance of knowing your smear result. There is a strong case to be made for women always to be sent a copy of their own smear result at the same time as it is sent to their doctor. It would result in many more anxious visits for explanations, but it would save lives.

As you have probably realised, there is much room for improvement in the way we test for cervical pre-cancer and the way in which tests are followed up. However, there are now developments in the offing which may change all that. In Chapter 11 we look to the future.

10

PSYCHOLOGICAL AND EMOTIONAL ASPECTS

The whole issue of cervical smears and cervical cancer is fraught with anxiety for many women. This is to a large extent due to their poor understanding of the purpose of cervical screening and the meaning of an abnormal smear. The fact that a cervical smear is often called a cancer smear only increases the confusion and worry that surround it.

The anxiety begins before a woman has even attended for a smear. Many women, especially older women, dislike and are frightened of having an internal examination. They also feel embarrassed at the thought that it may be performed by a male doctor. Women are often unaware that they are perfectly entitled to request a female doctor or nurse; if your general practitioner is a man, you are at liberty to ask to see a female partner in the practice, or even attend a different practice for smears and family planning advice.

There is a good deal of confusion about the symptoms of cervical cancer and pre-cancer. Women often think that if they have not noticed anything wrong themselves (such as vaginal discharge or pain) then everything must be all right and they do not need to have a smear. This is a fundamental misconception about both the purpose of screening and the symptoms of cervical cancer.

The whole point of having cervical smears is to detect pre-cancers, which have *no symptoms at all*. There is no way a woman can know that she has abnormal cells on her cervix. And there is also another side to the coin; the symptoms of cervical cancer, which are bleeding after intercourse and discharge, are very commonly produced by other harmless conditions. For example, a cervical erosion (see Chapter 3) is a common cause of bleeding after intercourse, and there are many vaginal infections which cause discharge but which have nothing to do with cancer. So, paradoxically, a woman who has symptoms may actually be worrying quite unnecessarily, while the woman with no symptoms who thinks nothing is wrong may be in danger.

Women who have passed through the menopause (change of life) sometimes think that, since their womb has no function any more, nothing at all is going to happen 'down there'. This is, of course, not true, but again it makes them feel they do not need to have smears.

Many older women, as well as some young women, feel that attending for a cervical smear in some way implies that they have been promiscuous. They have heard that cervical cancer is associated with promiscuity, and are worried that their families and friends will think they must have a 'past' if they are having smears. Hopefully, this attitude is changing as the role of male sexual behaviour in the incidence of cervical cancer is increasingly publicised. After all, even faithful husbands of 20 years duration are likely to have had other partners before they were married.

THE CERVICAL SMEAR ITSELF

Having the smear test can sometimes be a traumatic experience, which may affect a woman's acceptance of screening in the future. Much depends on the woman herself; if she is determined to expect the worst, her wishes are likely to be fulfilled. We have before stressed the importance of trying to be relaxed during the examination: if you are tense, it can be uncomfortable; you then become more tense and it becomes more uncomfortable; and so on, in a vicious circle. The doctor or nurse will be trying to put you at your ease as much as possible, and there is nothing to stop you having a stiff drink beforehand or doing some relaxation exercises if they help. Some doctors and nurses remember that warming the speculum beforehand (e.g. under warm water) will make the examination more comfortable for you. If they don't remember, you can always suggest it.

An unfortunate aspect of some clinics and surgeries is that medical and nursing staff walk in and out of the rooms during consultations. You do not necessarily know who they are, and this may well make you more anxious. After all, it is a very private part of your life and anatomy which is on display. Doctors and nurses in busy clinics can forget how embarrassing such interruptions are for the women being examined; the staff are so used to seeing women undressed that they hardly notice any more. This does not, however, make it any easier for you as an individual. Do not hesitate to remind them of your need for privacy; rooms have doors which can easily be locked for a few minutes.

WAITING FOR RESULTS

It is unfortunate that many clinics and doctors only notify women of an abnormal smear result. This is usually because they do not have enough clerical staff to send out a letter to every woman who has been for a test. However, this means that women often wait anxiously for months, thinking the next post may bring the dreaded letter. In addition, when they hear nothing, they may worry that the letter has in fact gone astray.

One of the ways round this is for you to leave a stamped addressed envelope to be placed in your records. When your result is filed, a copy can then be sent to you, with very little extra effort on the part of the clinic staff. Alternatively, find out roughly how long results take to come back and either make an appointment for a week later, or whatever, or drop in to find out your result – ask your doctor or clinic which they would prefer. Sometimes, they will give negative results over the phone, although it would be unusual for an abnormal result to be given in this way.

Whatever you do, do not sit around at home worrying about your result; find out for yourself what it is.

AN ABNORMAL SMEAR RESULT

An abnormal smear result often unleashes a fearsome combination of anxiety, guilt, resentment and anger in otherwise perfectly sensible women. It is our fervent hope that, by writing this book, we will have prevented or allayed some of these reactions.

In Chapter 2 we discussed the meaning and implications of an abnormal smear result. The vast majority of abnormal smears are due to pre-cancers which are completely and easily curable. However, it is our experience that many women immediately assume they are in imminent danger of dying from cervical cancer, and are therefore understandably distressed.

Once again, the stigma of sexually transmitted disease rears its ugly head. Some women feel 'dirty' and ashamed that their sexual behaviour has resulted in disease. Others feel they are being punished for something. When you think of all the taboos that even today surround sexual behaviour, it is not surprising that women end up feeling guilty and unclean.

They may well turn on their unsuspecting man to vent their anger. Many of these women have only had one or two partners in their lives, and naturally assume that it is the current one who is to blame. However, the wart virus (if we assume this is likely to be the major cause) can lie dormant in cells for a very long time – perhaps for years. It is therefore quite impossible to try and work out who had it in the first place – unless, of course, the woman has only ever had one partner. This resentment directed at the male partner can, in turn, make him feel guilty and rejected. It is not uncommon for relationships to break up after a woman has discovered she has an abnormal smear. Paradoxically, this is often detrimental to the woman herself, as she may need a supportive partner to help her at this stressful time.

In fact, many men do feel guilty, even without being reminded. They may have already heard about the 'high-risk male' through television or newspaper articles. Men are often seen in sexually transmitted disease clinics asking to be checked for warts in case they might infect their girlfriends or wives. It is very frustrating for them to be told that there is no way they can be given an unconditional all clear – there is always the possibility of microscopic infection, for which nothing can be done. And unfortunately, some men go along looking for confirmation that they have no visible warts; if this is given, without the caution that there might be a microscopic infection, they may go home and accuse their partner of being unfaithful, or tell her it is 'her fault'. Accusations from either partner are only hurtful and achieve nothing positive. It is far more useful for both partners to realise each others' fears and guilt and help each other through the experience.

The most important thing to do if you are informed of an abnormal smear is to discuss it fully with your doctor. Only then can you be sure of what is going on and feel less frightened of the future. Friends can be useful in letting you know of their experiences, but remember that they are not you and their smear result may have been different from yours.

THE EFFECT OF COLPOSCOPY AND LOCAL TREATMENT

In theory, if women attending colposcopy clinics were fully informed about the meaning of their smear result, they should not be anxious. However, even informed women often experience anxiety at the thought of the examination and what might be found.

The position you have to lie in during a colposcopy examination can be described, at best, as inelegant. Once again, relaxation is important, especially as the procedure will take longer than a smear. Do not hesitate to ask for privacy; it will aid the doctor, as well as yourself, if you are not continually tensing up because people are constantly opening the door. It is sometimes said that once you have had a baby you can never be embarrassed by inelegant positions again. This is, quite frankly, rubbish. For a start, having a baby is (one hopes) an experience which is expected to have a pleasant and rewarding outcome. Women therefore approach it in quite a different manner, and perceive it differently. In addition, they are often so tired and so glad to get it over that they have ceased to care about elegance and privacy. Lastly, the memory of the actual labour and delivery, like many painful and unpleasant experiences, fades, and therefore cannot be readily drawn on for comparison. So do not let yourself be made to feel inadequate by this kind of statement, even though it may be well meant.

Although you will usually be given some idea of the likely result of your colposcopy examination, you will again have to wait several weeks for the full result while the biopsies are looked at in the laboratory. This is inevitable; no matter how experienced the doctor, he or she cannot guarantee 100 per cent accuracy in diagnosis from the examination alone, so the full result has to include the report on the biopsies.

So here you are, waiting anxiously once again. Ideally, you should be given a follow-up appointment to see your colposcopist in order to discuss the results and what needs to be done next. Unfortunately, many such doctors are just too busy for this to happen. They may explain the possibilities to you at your initial visit, and then simply send you another appointment for whatever examination or treatment is appropriate. This works reasonably well in most cases; remember that the vast majority of abnormalities are only pre-cancers, and the actual degree of pre-cancer is not very important once a definite assessment has been made. The treatment is much the same for all of them, so the only thing which may vary is the speed with which treatment is given; obviously, higher degrees of pre-cancer will be given priority over milder ones.

Usually, if the results are very different from the initial impression during the colposcopy, you will be given an appointment to come back and discuss them. However, they can be just as easily better as worse than first thought, so do not immediately assume the worst.

TREATMENT

Now we come to the treatment. Several months are likely to have elapsed since your original smear result. For some women this is an advantage, as it gives them time to settle their thoughts and anxieties, and approach the whole issue with greater equanimity. However, the waiting makes other women increasingly nervous. Tensions can build up at home, concentrating on a job can be difficult, and so on. If you were already an anxious or unhappy person before all this happened, you are much more likely to have difficulty coping with this experience. Seek help. There is little point in struggling on by yourself when a little counselling may be all that is needed.

The majority of women find the actual treatment itself to be far less dreadful and painful than they thought. They are therefore usually relieved that it is all over, and with so little fuss. However, the thought that part of their cervix has had to be destroyed leaves many women with psychological and psychosexual problems. A recent study compared women who had abnormal smears with those who had come into contact with a different sexually transmitted disease, non-specific urethritis. The study looked at features such as interest in sex, feelings towards the partner, pain during sex and satisfaction with sex. Women who had an abnormal smear necessitating colposcopy and treatment were found to have far more negative feelings towards sex than those who knew their partners had non-specific urethritis and were treated for it themselves.

Interestingly, women who knew their partners had penile warts, but who themselves had a normal cervical smear, did not react in this negative fashion. Although they knew they had come into contact with a risk factor, and the connotations were presumably much the same, psychologically they did not seem to be affected any more than women whose partners had non-specific urethritis.

It is also interesting that it did not seem to be the abnormal smear itself which was associated with psychosexual problems. No change in attitude was noted from the time the women knew their smear was abnormal to the time they had their colposcopy, even though, in many cases, this interval amounted to several months. However, their attitudes changed significantly *after* they had had colposcopy and treatment. They showed loss of interest in sex, felt hostile towards their partner, did not enjoy sex as much as before, and often said they experienced pain during intercourse.

Now, of course, these feelings are often related to one another, and may be related most of all to the woman's anxiety. For example, a woman who is feeling anxious about her cervix may well be worried about having sex. She is therefore not very relaxed during intercourse and does not find the experience as pleasant and satisfying as before. Anxiety about her sexual performance may then be added to her other worries. The next time she has sex she will therefore be twice as anxious as before, and will thus be more tense, find it more uncomfortable and even less pleasant. A vicious circle soon develops, as a result of which she is likely to feel that it is preferable not to have sex at all and avoid the issue altogether.

The results of this study are very worrying. Cervical pre-cancer is increasingly being found in young women. They may not yet have found a stable relationship, or started their family. It is obvious from this research that they are being placed at a considerable disadvantage in future relationships, and may develop a variety of psychosexual problems which may both hinder the formation of a relationship or harm an existing one.

These women and their partners need help. However, psychosexual counselling is not always easy to come by. It would be very useful if counselling services could be developed in colposcopy clinics to help what is bound to be a growing problem. Indeed, it could be argued that counselling should become a routine part of the whole treatment process; after all, prevention is better than cure. At present, counselling is usually limited to specialised units. A few useful addresses have been included in the appendix on page 125, and your family planning clinic or general practitioner may be able to give you further advice on local facilities.

CANCER

There can be few pieces of news which are worse to give or receive than a diagnosis of cancer. The person receiving it sees before them a bleak future of pain, suffering and, ultimately, death. The person giving it knows this and feels a mixture of sympathy, sorrow and guilt, as though it were somehow their fault and that it is somehow unfair that they are healthy. It is important to realise that the families of the affected person will also have feelings of guilt, of sorrow and of helplessness. Sometimes this helplessness turns into hostility directed at the person giving the news, or even towards the woman herself. A great deal of understanding on all sides is therefore required at such a difficult time.

A great deal may be said at the time the diagnosis is given, but it is unlikely that the woman or her family will take much in. It is therefore important that a second appointment is made, soon after the first, at which the whole issue is discussed again. It is likely that, by this time, both the woman and her family will have many questions which need to be answered.

It is worth bearing in mind, if you find yourself in this unhappy position, that the doctor who sees you is only a human being. It is very unlikely that he or she has had any training in counselling techniques; it is somehow expected that these will be 'picked up' on the way. The doctor may therefore be feeling very awkward and may not really know what to say or how to say it, despite wanting to be as sympathetic and helpful as possible. However, do not feel inhibited from asking questions; it is often easier in such situations for the doctor to answer questions than to try and think what a woman might want or need to know.

The association of cervical cancer with sex makes some women feel very guilty. This is particularly marked in women who have had abortions or extra-marital affairs. They may feel they are being punished for what they have done. Young women who have not had children may feel both cheated and punished, and may have strong feelings of both guilt and resentment. Sometimes, these women, who feel they have 'got what they deserve', become deceptively good, compliant patients. It is as if they feel they may get a reprieve for good behaviour. These women need counselling; such bargaining is likely to lead only to disappointment and further psychological problems.

HYSTERECTOMY

The treatment of cancer often requires a hysterectomy (removal of the womb – or uterus). Many women find this daunting and disturbing. The uterus is often perceived as the essence of a woman's femininity; without it, she may feel she is no longer a 'complete' woman. Also, periods are sometimes felt to be a 'cleansing of the system', without which poisons of some kind will accumulate in the body. If the ovaries are to be removed as well, she may feel she will age prematurely.

It can take a great deal of explaining to persuade a woman that the uterus is nothing more than a box used to package a baby. It has no other function. The blood which is shed each month is only the lining of the uterus, which has thickened during the cycle in preparation for a fertilised egg which never materialised. Periods have no other meaning or function. Ovaries produce hormones and eggs, but the hormones can easily be replaced by synthetic ones, with no noticeable change in effect.

Hysterectomy involves a considerable change in a woman's

self-image. For a start, she will no longer be capable of having children. Some women will accept this with relief, as they will no longer need to worry about contraception. They may even find their sex life improves when this anxiety is removed. However, other women find the idea of sex with no possibility of conception difficult. All methods of contraception have a failure rate, no matter how small; this element of risk may be crucial for some women to enjoy sex. They may therefore lose interest in sex after a hysterectomy. Some women may even feel they have been mutilated by the operation, and may feel they are now deformed, despite their normal outward appearance. They may worry that they will not be able to have sex normally as a result of the operation. This, of course, can become a self-fulfilling prophecy, as the anxiety interferes with sexual response, thus with enjoyment, and so on.

In fact a hysterectomy should make very little or no difference to a woman's life, including her sex life. During the weeks following the operation she will, of course, feel tired, perhaps weak. Women often say it takes about two months before they feel themselves again. However, it is important that they should resume their sex lives sooner rather than later; the later they leave it the more likely they are to experience difficulty when restarting.

The role of a supportive partner cannot be emphasised enough. He can do a great deal to allay her fears that she will no longer be attractive or feminine. Even when actual intercourse is impossible, he can show his affection for her in other ways, thus maintaining her confidence in herself and in their relationship.

Once again, the pre-existing emotional state of the woman and the stability of the relationship are important factors in determining how she will cope following the operation. Women who tend towards depression and anxiety in normal life are more likely to suffer after the operation. Similarly, an already unstable relationship may dissolve completely under the strain.

Sometimes, even being pronounced cured can be stressful. A woman may have channelled all her strength and emotion into coping with the knowledge and reality of cancer, and it may be difficult to readjust to being a normal, healthy person. Again, understanding and help from family and friends is important in making the adjustment successfully.

RADIOTHERAPY

Many people are frightened of radiation, and therefore fear this treatment almost as much as the disease itself. The fact that treatment goes on for several weeks, and is often accompanied by ill-health, does not help in coping with it emotionally. Extensive counselling is therefore needed, both to discuss initial fears and to cope with side effects during and after treatment.

Unfortunately, radiotherapy causes the tissues in the pelvis to stiffen, or fibrose, and this does lead to problems during sex. Women and their partners will need advice as to positions which will be most comfortable; these are likely to be those in which deep penetration does not occur, at least initially. Radiotherapy also interferes with the function of the ovaries, resulting in a lack of oestrogen. This can, and should be, replaced with synthetic hormones (hormone replacement therapy). Not only will this help the woman psychologically, but it actually helps in the healing of the tissues.

One of the side effects which occurs during treatment is that the woman may notice vaginal discharge and bleeding, especially after intercourse. This is particularly alarming, as these are likely to be the very symptoms she had before the diagnosis of cancer was made. It is important to understand that they are simply a side effect, and not signs of things getting worse.

Some people think that they become dangerous to others while receiving radiation, which may add to negative feelings they already have about themselves. It is only true, and then usually for only a short time, if a source of radiation is actually placed within the body. It certainly does not apply to external radiation treatment; you do not glow in the dark afterwards.

Radiotherapy is often viewed with disappointment when compared to surgery – it is nice to feel that the cancer has been actually cut out and taken away. This is not the case with radiotherapy, but it is important to remember that it can still result in a cure.

RADICAL SURGERY AND CHEMOTHERAPY

These really are outside the scope of this book. Both forms of treatment are a last resort and it is not surprising, therefore, that the women who receive them are likely to be depressed and anxious. As always, counselling is very important in helping women and their families cope. Comprehensive information as to what to expect and what can be done about side effects is essential.

IN SUMMARY

You may have noticed that throughout this chapter we have constantly referred to the psychosexual problems which may occur following treatment of pre-cancer or cancer. You may be thinking 'Surely sex is the last thing on a woman's mind when she finds she has a potentially life-threatening condition?'

This is absolutely true. At first, all she is interested in is being cured. However, life has to go on, and since pre-cancer, at least, is completely curable, life should go on as it did before. And even a woman with cancer may have many potentially rewarding years of life ahead of her.

A woman's self-image is often dependent greatly on her perception of how she functions as a woman. This also means that the relationship she has with her partner will be crucial in deciding how she will cope with her condition and her future life. This is not to say that the relationship always has to be successful; sometimes the breakdown of an unsatisfactory or destructive relationship may have a positive effect on her attitude to the future. It is important that both the woman concerned and her doctors recognise that she and her partner may need counselling, both psychological and psychosexual, even though that need may not be immediately apparent to any of them.

11

THE FUTURE

As we have seen, the deficiencies of the cervical smear test are many, and furthermore they are difficult to eradicate. Errors can occur in the technique of taking the smear, in its interpretation at the laboratory, and in its inherent accuracy in predicting the degree of abnormality present.

The technical accuracy of smears can be improved by using a better design of spatula, or an endocervical brush. These have been discussed in more detail in Chapters 1, 3 and 9.

THE FREE RADICAL METHOD

Interpretation of smears at present allows too much room for human error (the reasons for this have been discussed in Chapter 9). The only real way in which laboratory error can be minimised is by using an automated process, and so far it has not been possible to read smear slides by machine. However, a new method of processing smears is undergoing trials; if these continue to be successful it could dispense with cytology altogether.

The method relies on measuring the concentrations of two chemicals on the cell surface. Both are types of linoleic acid, a chemical which forms part of the cell structure. Normal cells have mostly type 1 linoleic acid, but abnormal cells have been shown to have more of type 2. Initial tests have shown that it is actually possible to predict the degree of abnormality from the amount of type 2 linoleic acid present, i.e. the more type 2 linoleic acid there is, the greater the abnormality. It is thought that abnormal cells produce substances called free radicals which react with type 1 linoleic acid and turn it into type 2.

If we were to measure the differences in the very small concentrations of types 1 and 2 linoleic acid found on the cervical cells collected from a smear, there would undoubtedly be unacceptable levels of inaccuracy. Instead, therefore, we measure the ratio of concentration of type 1 to type 2. In this way, the actual number of cells present does not matter.

So far the test has a sensitivity of between 80 and 90 per cent. This means it has a false negative rate (in the presence of abnormal cells) of between 10 and 20 per cent, compared with a false negative rate of up to 50 per cent for the ordinary smear. Although it would obviously be good if the accuracy could be improved still further, this method has one enormous advantage over the ordinary smear; it can be completely automated. The smear is taken as usual, but then, instead of wiping the spatula onto a slide, it is shaken in a bottle of special solution. The bottle is subsequently transported to a laboratory, where a special machine works out the concentrations. The machine can analyse a large number of samples at the same time, so the process is quick, cheap and not subject to human error. It certainly sounds very promising, but is still in its early stages. More trials need to be done before it can be widely adopted.

Research is also looking into a second technique which could be automated. This involves staining the DNA in the cells on a smear and measuring its optical density. The greater the density, the greater the abnormality. This work is also still at a very early stage, but looks promising.

CERVICOGRAPHY

The problem of the high false negative rate of smears could be almost completely eradicated if the smear test was used in conjunction with a new screening method called cervicography.

Cervicography was developed in 1981 by a gynaecologist in the United States. He was worried by the inaccuracy of the smear test when he compared it with his findings at colposcopy. Colposcopy was so obviously better at detecting abnormalities, but the idea of using it as a screening method was out of the question; the equipment is very expensive, the examination is time consuming, and there simply aren't enough doctors who are trained in this specialist technique.

This particular gynaecologist also happened to be a former professional photographer. It occurred to him that if a photograph of the cervix could be taken at the same time as the smear, it would be a great help in improving accuracy. Taking photographs using the colposcope was already an established technique. It was very useful for keeping records of abnormalities as well as for teaching purposes; the abnormal areas showed up well on a photograph and could therefore be discussed at lectures and meetings, without the need for the woman in question to be present. This obviously spared her the embarrassment and was much more practical.

Taking photographs through a colposcope, however, is almost as difficult as the colposcopy itself – indeed, as most doctors are only just about able to work an instamatic camera, the quality of their pictures using a complicated camera and focusing system can leave a great deal to be desired. Being both a gynaecologist and a photographer, he realised that what was needed was a method which would allow photographs of the cervix to be taken by doctors who were trained neither in colposcopy nor in photography. The colposcope itself provides a light source; if this was not present, the camera would have to have a flash unit attached. The colposcope also provides magnification to help see abnormal areas; however, this means that if you are not an expert you may photograph the wrong area, or miss an important section. It was therefore concluded that what was needed was a photograph of the entire cervix, which was of such good quality that it could be magnified, i.e. enlarged massively, later. A good transparency (slide) will do this. The single most important technical feature of a good-quality photograph is that it should be in focus – so the focusing had to be made foolproof. What he came up with was the cerviscope.

The cerviscope is basically a 35 mm camera with a built-in flash and a fixed focus. The exposure and flash are automatically controlled. All the operator has to do is press a button. The photograph, or cervicogram as it is called, is taken at the time of an ordinary vaginal examination. A speculum is inserted, just as for a smear. The cervix is wiped with a little acetic acid, as in colposcopy; this makes any abnormal areas show up white. A photograph is then taken of the whole cervix, using the cerviscope. As you can see in the illustration on the next page, all the doctor or nurse has to do is point the

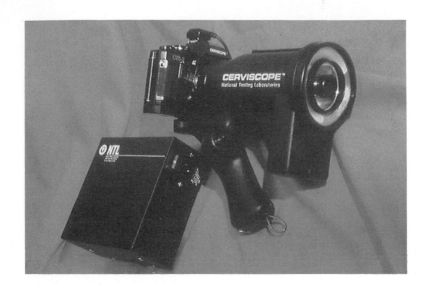

Cerviscope.

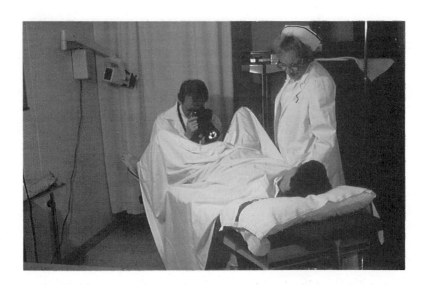

Cervicography in progress.

cerviscope in the direction of the cervix, looking through the speculum. The procedure is then repeated using the iodine stain, as a double check. The whole thing only takes a couple of minutes. And the beauty of the system is that it requires absolutely no training, other than that of performing a speculum examination. It also requires no equipment, apart from the camera itself. Therefore any doctor, and many nurses, can do it.

Once the photograph has been taken it is processed and then sent to an expert colposcopist for evaluation. He can project the slides on a screen and thus gets a very large picture of the cervix, comparable to the view at colposcopy. Being an expert, he can quickly tell if there is any abnormality present, and can also make a reasonably accurate estimate of the actual degree of abnormality. His report is then sent back to the doctor who took the picture, just like a smear result.

This method has been shown to have a false negative rate of only about 3 per cent. However, it does have a false positive rate of about 16 per cent; this means that in 16 per cent of cases women will be called up for colposcopy when, in fact,

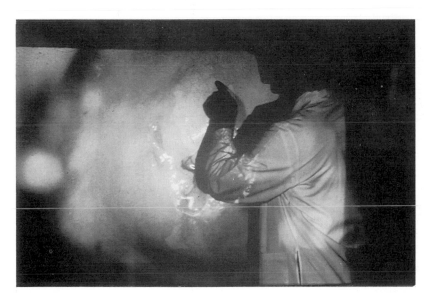

Cervicogram.

their cervix is normal. This is undesirable, because of the unnecessary anxiety which is caused; also, of course, it is a waste of everyone's time.

Why is there such a high false positive rate? Well, basically it is because the person assessing the picture is always likely to err on the side of caution. If he sees anything which looks even faintly abnormal he will want a better look – when looking at a photograph you cannot, after all, move the cervix around to get a better view. However, it is surely preferable to call up a few women unnecessarily than to miss large numbers of abnormalities, as happens with the smear.

Cervicography has one further limitation. It cannot show up any abnormalities which are hidden from an ordinary face-on view. This means that an abnormality which is in the endocervical canal will be missed. For this reason, it should be used in conjunction with, and not as a replacement for, the cervical smear. A useful system might be to take only an endocervical smear, using the cytobrush, in addition to the cervicogram. That way, if the photograph showed nothing but the smear was abnormal, it would be obvious that the abnormality had to be in the endocervical canal. This method should almost completely eliminate false negatives.

A useful feature of cervicography is that a print can be made from the slide and kept in the woman's notes. This is good because it provides a permanent record of the appearance of her cervix at that time, and can be used for comparison during future examinations. It also means the woman herself can see what is wrong with her cervix, and exactly how big any area of abnormality is. It is much easier to grasp such concepts if there is something visual to back up the information.

Cervicography is already in use in the United States, and is gradually filtering through into the rest of the world. The cerviscopes are quite expensive, which is a problem if it is to be widely used. In addition, there are administrative difficulties in setting up the reporting service in some countries. However, the initial outlay should be offset in the long run by the reduction in cervical cancer achieved. This, of course, applies to any successful screening method; the costs of looking after women with cervical cancer are immense compared with treatment at the pre-cancerous stage.

Another possible use of the technique is being tried in London. Women who have a very mildly abnormal smear are offered cervicography in order to assess more accurately and rapidly the degree, if any, of their abnormality. The photographs are taken by nurses, who also counsel the women beforehand. In this way, women are reassured, both in terms of the rapidity of diagnosis and by talking to an informed counsellor about their smear.

THE WART VIRUS

In Chapter 8, we looked at the evidence linking the human papilloma virus (HPV or wart virus) with cervical cancer. One of the interesting findings has been that only a small number of the 40 or so types of HPV are actually linked with cervical cancer itself. So, although types 6 and 11 are commonly found in genital warts and in the milder forms of cervical pre-cancer, it is types 16 and 18 which are usually found in cervical cancer tissue.

Cervical pre-cancer is becoming increasingly common. In addition, in terms of numbers, there is far more mild dyskaryosis (dysplasia) than anything else. A proportion of these very mild cell changes will get better on their own in time, and a certain number will simply stay the same. However, about a third will go on to severe dyskaryosis and from there to cancer. It is because we do not know which category an individual woman will fall into that we have to treat everyone the same. If we could tell which type of HPV was present in the cells, we would be able to predict the outcome much more accurately. For example, a woman whose smear shows mild dyskaryosis with only HPV types 6 or 11 present is unlikely to get cancer. She should simply have regular testing, to make sure the pre-cancer is not progressing and to check that no new HPV types have appeared. However, the women with mild dyskaryosis who has HPV types 16 or 18 in the cells is at much greater risk of progressing to cancer. She should therefore be offered treatment.

Methods of testing cells for the HPV types they contain already exist. In very general terms it is done by looking at the DNA present in the nucleus of the cell; each virus has its own particular type of DNA, which is like a fingerprint. However, because it is a specialised and expensive technique, only large hospitals which are interested in research have the necessary laboratory facilities. This means that it would be very impractical to try and use it for mass screening at present.

SOLVING THE MANPOWER SHORTAGE

There is a worldwide shortage of colposcopy clinics and doctors trained in the specialty. If, as is predicted, there continues to be an increase in cervical cancer and pre-cancer, this shortage is likely to become acute. At present, the vast majority of colposcopists are hospital gynaecologists. To become a hospital gynaecologist takes about 15 years and involves training in all aspects of obstetrics and gynaecology. However, any doctor who has some basic gynaecological experience can be trained to perform colposcopy. It therefore makes very good sense for doctors in related specialties, such as genito-urinary medicine and family planning, to become at least part-time colposcopists. Large numbers of women have their smears taken in such clinics; it is likely to be more pleasant for them to have colposcopy performed in a familiar setting, perhaps by a doctor they already know, and would also provide job satisfaction for the doctors involved. Another advantage is that both genito-urinary medicine clinics and many family planning clinics are either physically attached to or have close links with the local major hospital. This is important, because there needs to be both close liaison and trust between those who are performing the colposcopies and the hospital gynaecologists. After all, it is the gynaecologists who will take over if treatment is necessary, and who may need to be called in to give a second opinion. It is also important that the clinics and the hospital should use the same cytology and histopathology laboratories. As we mentioned in Chapter 10, there is often considerable variation in the way smears are reported. It is therefore sensible to try and maintain a consistent approach when a patient moves between clinics and the hospital.

For such a scheme to work, it is imperative that there is agreement between the clinics performing colposcopy and the gynaecologists. There is no point in a woman having a colposcopy performed in her clinic, only to be told it will have to be done again at the hospital because the gynaecologists are not willing to trust the findings. This can actually be detrimental to her case, as she will have had a biopsy taken in the clinic, which may make a subsequent colposcopy much more difficult to interpret. For this reason, it is in general unwise for individual doctors to try and set up a colposcopy service on their own, unless they are also competent and have the facilities to carry out the necessary treatments.

A useful arrangement, which suits both sides, is for the gynaecologists to train individual doctors from local clinics. In this way the gynaecologists can be satisfied of the level of competence in the clinics, and will therefore have confidence in their management. It also helps tremendously in communication if people have met each other.

This trend towards colposcopy outside hospital gynaecology departments is bound to continue, and should benefit women by decreasing their waiting time and lessening their anxiety over the procedure.

CONCLUSION

The future holds many exciting new prospects in this field of medicine. We have only been able to discuss a few of them in this book, and more are appearing all the time. However, whatever method of screening is used, the most important thing is for you to make sure you have made use of it. Cervical cancer is completely preventable – and the person best able to prevent it is you.

FURTHER READING

Your Smear Test
Graham H. Barker
Adamson Books, London

Hysterectomy: What It Is, and How To Cope With It Successfully
Suzie Hayman
Sheldon Press, London

The Pill
John Guillebaud
Oxford University Press

Contraception: Your Questions Answered
John Guillebaud
Churchill Livingstone, London

Your Body: A Woman's Guide To Her Sexual Health
Thorsons, Wellingborough, Northamptonshire

Women's Health Guide: An Illustrated Handbook of the Female Body
Angela Mills
Windward

Do-It-Yourself Psychotherapy
Martin Shepard
Macdonald Optima, London

The Book of Love
Dr David Delvin
New English Library, London

Sexually Transmitted Diseases: The Facts
David Barlow
Oxford University Press

Below the Belt: A Woman's Guide to Genito-Urinary Infections
Denise Winn
Macdonald Optima, London

Private Parts: A Health Book for Men
Dr Yosh Taguchi
Macdonald Optima, London

Your Cancer, Your Life
Dr Trish Reynolds
Macdonald Optima, London

USEFUL ADDRESSES/ ORGANISATIONS

UK
The Health Education Authority
78 New Oxford St
London WC1A 1AH
01-631 0930
Provides information and leaflets on many aspects of health and screening.

Scottish Health Education Group
Woodburn House
Canaan Lane
Edinburgh EH10 4SG
031-447 8044
Similar to the above.

The Family Planning Association
27–35 Mortimer St
London W1N 7RJ
01-636 7866
Gives advice on all aspects of family planning, sexual problems, etc. A good source of information about other clinics and services available throughout the United Kingdom. They also have free leaflets on many topics.

Margaret Pyke Centre for Study and Training in Family Planning
15 Bateman's Buildings
Soho Square
London W1V 5TW
01-734 9351
The largest centre in Europe, dealing with all aspects of family planning, counselling and screening.

Brook Advisory Centres (head office)
233 Tottenham Court Rd
London W1
01-323 1522/01-580 2991
Specialise in young people's problems (under 24). Provide family planning screening services and counselling.

British Association for Counselling
37A Sheep St
Rugby
Warwickshire CV21 3BX
0788 78328
Useful source of nationwide information about clinics which provide counselling.

National Marriage Guidance Council (head office)
Herbert Gray College
Little Church St
Rugby
Warwickshire CV21 3AP
0788 73241
Nationwide network of clinics providing psychosexual and marriage guidance counselling.

Association of Sexual and Marital Therapists
PO Box 62
Sheffield S10 3TS

Sexually transmitted disease clinics
Most large hospitals have one, or will be able to tell you where the nearest one is.

The Herpes Association
39 North Rd
London N6
01-609 9061

Terence Higgins Trust
BM AIDS
London WC1N 3XX
01-833 2971
01-278 8745
Helpline 01-833 2971
Information, support groups and counselling about AIDS.

Hysterectomy Support Group
11 Henryson Rd
London SE4 1HL
01-690 5987
Self-help organisation for women who have had, or are going
to have, a hysterectomy.

Women's Health Concern
17 Earl's Terrace
London W8 6LP
01-602 6669
Information about all aspects of women's health.

The Women's National Cancer Control Campaign
1 South Audley St
London W1Y 5D
01-499 7532/4

Women Against Cervical Cancer (WACC)
86 Beaufort St
London SW3 6BU
01-352 1440

Women's Health Information Centre (WHIC)
52 Featherstone St
London EC1
01-251 6580

British Association of Cancer United Patients (BACUP)
121–123 Charterhouse St
London EC1M 6AA
01-608 1661

The Patients' Association
Room 33, 18 Charing Cross Rd
London WC2
01-240 0671

The Marie Curie Foundation
28 Belgrave Square
London SW1X 8BG
01-235 3325

Private screening clinics

Marie Stopes House
The Well Woman Centre
108 Whitfield St
London W1
01-388 0662/2585

Marie Stopes Centre
10 Queen Square
Leeds LS2 8AJ
0532 440685

Marie Stopes Centre
1 Police St
Manchester M2 7LQ
061-832 4250

PPP Female Health Screening
99 New Cavendish St
London W1M 7FQ
01-637 8941

BUPA Women's Unit
300 Gray's Inn Rd
London WC1
01-837 6484

Medical Express
Chapel Place
Oxford St
London W1
01-499 1991

Hanway Clinic (family planning, cervical smears, colposcopy,
sexually transmitted disease)
1 Hanway Place
London W1P 9DF
01-636 0366

Regent's Park Clinic (sexually transmitted disease)
184 Gloucester Place
London NW1 6DS
01-402 2208

EIRE

Irish Family Planning Clinic
Cathal Brugha Street Clinic
Dublin 1
Dublin 727276/727363
Provides a similar service to the FPA within the confines of
Irish law.

UNITED STATES

Planned Parenthood Federation of America (head office)
2010 Massachusetts Avenue
NW Suite 500
Washington DC 20036
202 785 3351

Western region:
333 Broadway
3rd Floor
San Francisco
California 94133
415 956 8856

Southern region:
3030 Peachtree Road
NW Room 303
Atlanta
Georgia 30305

Northern region:
2625 Butterfield Rd
Oak Brook
Illinois 60521
312 986 9270

AUSTRALIA

Australian Federation of FPAs
Suite 603
6th Floor
Roden Cutler House
24 Campbell St
Sydney
NSW 2000

NEW ZEALAND

The New Zealand FPA Inc.
PO Box 68200
214 Karangahape
Newton
Auckland

SOUTH AFRICA

FPA of South Africa
412 York House
46 Kerk St
Johannesburg 2001

INDEX

abnormal smear result 15–19, 103–105
acetic acid 41, 86
actinomyces 32–4
acyclovir 88
adolescence 75–6
antibiotics 29
antibodies 80
antitrypsin 76
anxiety 101–112
atrophy 37
Ayres' spatula 9

barrier contraception 74
basement membrane 5
biopsy 41–2; *see also* cone biopsy
bleomycin 89

cancer: cervical 6, 59–67; reactions to diagnosis 108–109
candida 28–30
carcinoma in situ 18
cells 5
Cervex brush 25
cervical: cancer 6, 59–67; erosion 25; intra-epithelial neoplasia 19
cervicography 21, 114–19
chemotherapy 66, 111–12
CIN classification *see* cervical intra-epithelial neoplasia
circumcision 73–4
CMV *see* cytomegalovirus
cohort effect 92

cold coagulation 48
colposcope 41
colposcopy 20–21, 36, 39–43, 99–100, 105–106
cone biopsy 42, 53–7
counselling 106
cryoprobe 47
cryotherapy 26, 47, 89
cystoscopy 63
cytobrush 7, 9, 95
cytology 10
cytomegalovirus 81–2
cytotoxic drugs 66

death rate 91
degrees of cancer 60–61
deoxyribonucleic acid 79–80
DNA *see* deoxyribonucleic acid
dyskariosis 18, 19, 98
dysplasia 17–18, 76, 98
dysplastic cells 17

ectropion 25–6
electrodiathermy 47–8
endocervical cells 13, 23–5
erosion, cervical 25–6
external radiotherapy 65

Flagyl *see* metronidazole
5 fluorouracil 89
free radical smear interpretation 113–14

gardnerella 27–8
genital warts 84–90
guilt 104

herpes simplex virus 82–3
high-risk male 72, 86
hormone: deficiency 59; replacement therapy 66
HPV *see* human papilloma virus
HSV *see* herpes simplex virus
human papilloma virus 83–90, 119
hysterectomy 57, 64–5, 109–110

immune system 87
Immunovir *see* inosine pranobex
inflammatory smear 34–7
inosine pranobex 90
internal radiotherapy 65
intra-uterine contraceptive devices 32–4
intravenous: pyelogram 63; urogram 63
invasive cancer 63–4
iodine 41
IUD *see* intra-uterine contraceptive device
IVP *see* intravenous pyelogram
IVU *see* intravenous urogram

koilocytes 85

lactobacilli 29
laser: cone biopsy 56; treatment 49–51; wart therapy 89
Lerners spatula 9

Meig's hysterectomy 64
menopause 37, 57, 59, 64, 66, 102
metronidazole 28, 32
microinvasion 62–3
mini-pill *see* progestogen only pill
monilia *see* candida

Nabothian follicles 6
negative test result 23–5, 96
neoplasia 19

oestrogen 37
os, external and internal 1

Pap test *see* Papanicolaou smear
Papanicolaou smear 6
papilloma 83–90
podophyllum 89
POP *see* progestogen only pill
positive smear 15–19
pre-cancerous lesions 45
pregnancy 45, 52, 75
progestogen only pill 74

protozoan 31
psychosexual problems 106–107

radical surgery 66–7, 111–12
radiotherapy 65–6, 111
record cards 97
report form 10–14
ribonucleic acid 79–80
RNA *see* ribonucleic acid

screening programmes 94
sexual behaviour 69–73
smegma 73
smoking 74, 87, 88
social class 70
spatula 7, 8, 9
special clinics 27
speculum 6–7, 41, 102
squamous: cells 5, 86–7; -columnar junction 6; metaplasia 15, 76
surgical cone biopsy 54–5

test results 103–105, 106
thrush *see* candida
transformation zone 5, 15, 86
trichloracetic acid 89
trichomonas vaginalis 31–2
trypsin 76
TV *see* trichomonas vaginalis

uterus 1

vagina 5
viruses 76–7, 79–90

warts 83–90, 119
Wertheim's hysterectomy 64
womb *see* uterus